Detox Drink Recipes to Make at Home

Quick and Easy Detoxification Drinks

BY: Ivy Hope

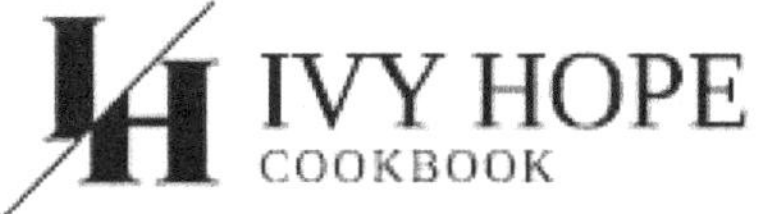

Copyright/License Page

Please don't reproduce this book. It means you are not allowed to make any type of copy (print or electronic), sell, publish, disseminate or distribute. Only people who have written permission from the author are allowed to do so.

This book is written by the author taking all precautions that the content is true and helpful. However, the reader needs to be careful about his/her action. If anything happens due to the reader's actions the author won't be taken as responsible.

Table of Contents

Introduction

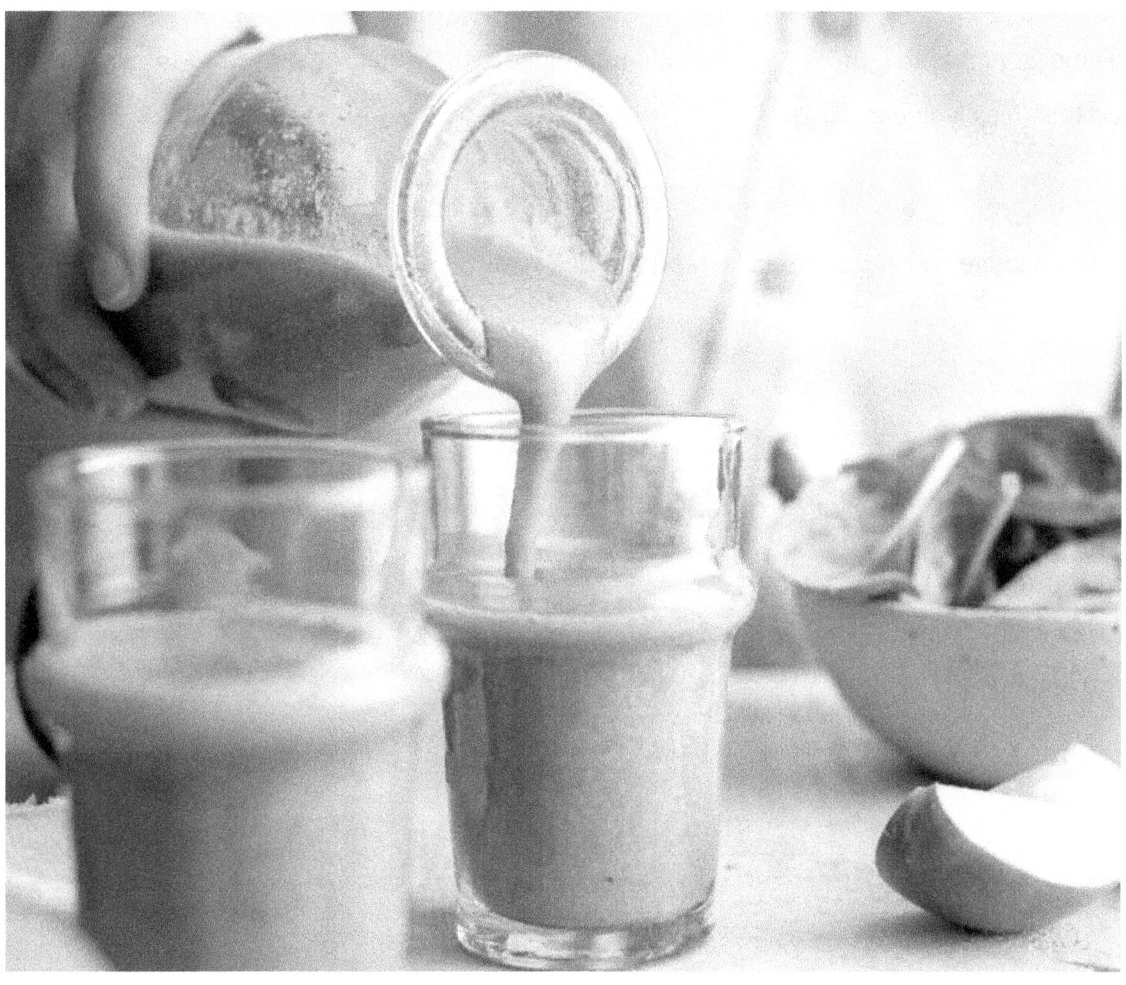

Detoxification helps you to have a healthy body and mind. We all need to remove the bad toxins from our bodies. When detoxing, I have found it to be easier with juices. You can make juices within a couple of minutes.

Once you start the detoxification process, you will feel much better. Your hair will look better, the extra pounds will go away (a little at a time), the skin will look younger, and newer. That's only a few positive outcomes of detoxing the body.

The best part is the juices can be made in a blender or a juicer. No need to think I cannot do this. Yes, you can.

Make sure you use 100% organic fruits and vegetables in your juices. Definitely, we don't need to add any chemicals to our bodies again.

2-year-old Kid-Friendly Ginger-Snap

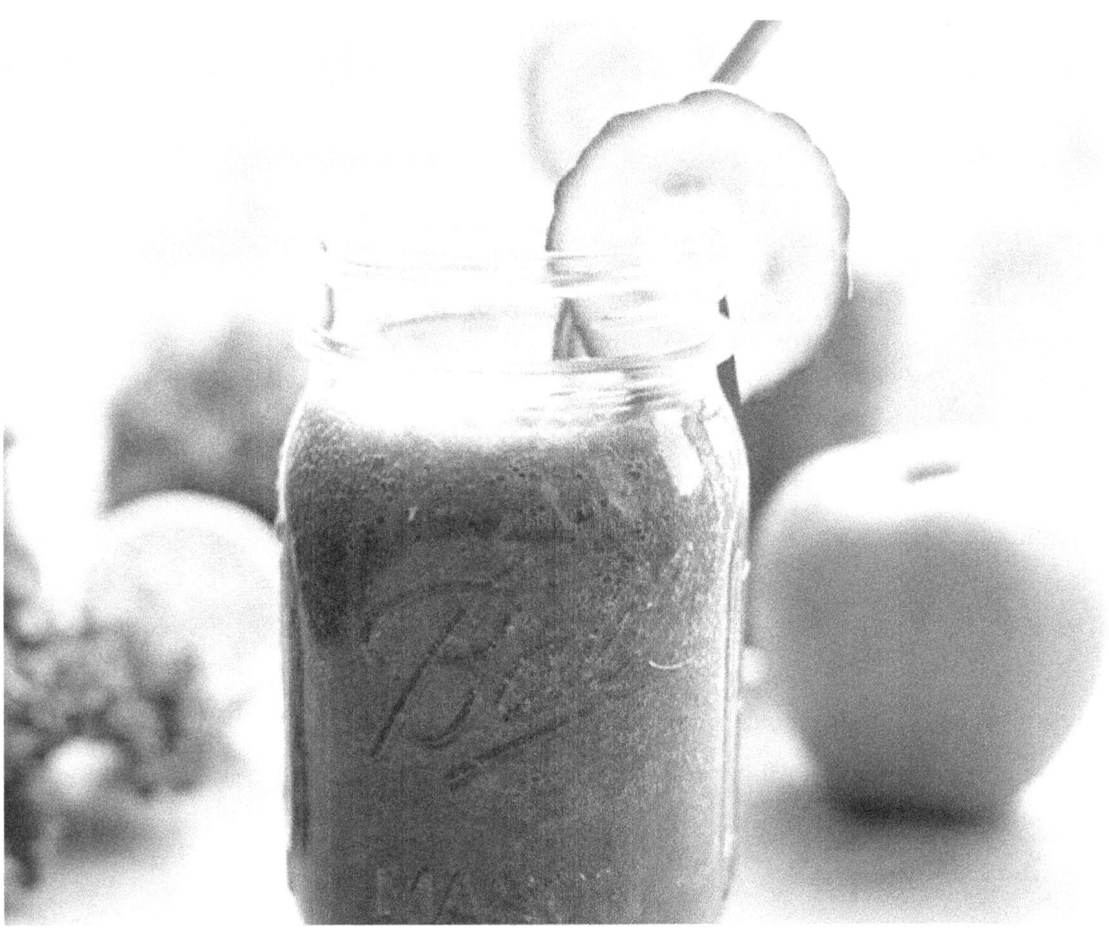

From time to time, a child also needs to have the toxins removed from the body. What you might be thinking. Have you noticed your child getting sick more than normal? Maybe, they are feeling sleepy or worn out. It's time to detox.

Makes 2 cups (8-ounces)

Serving: 1/2 cup (4-ounces)

Ingredients:

- 2 Organic medium Kiwi
- 1/4 Inch of fresh Ginger
- 2 Organic Celery Stalks
- 1 Organic Lemon Peeled
- 1 Medium organic cucumber
- 1 Small Organic Green Apple

Directions:

Using your blender, place the ingredients in the cup and blend on high for 1 minute or until smooth.

TIP:

I myself give my children ½ cup 1 hour before each meal. This gives the juice time to get into the body. Please don't think this juice is for replacing meals. It should never replace a meal.

Beet-a-full Day!

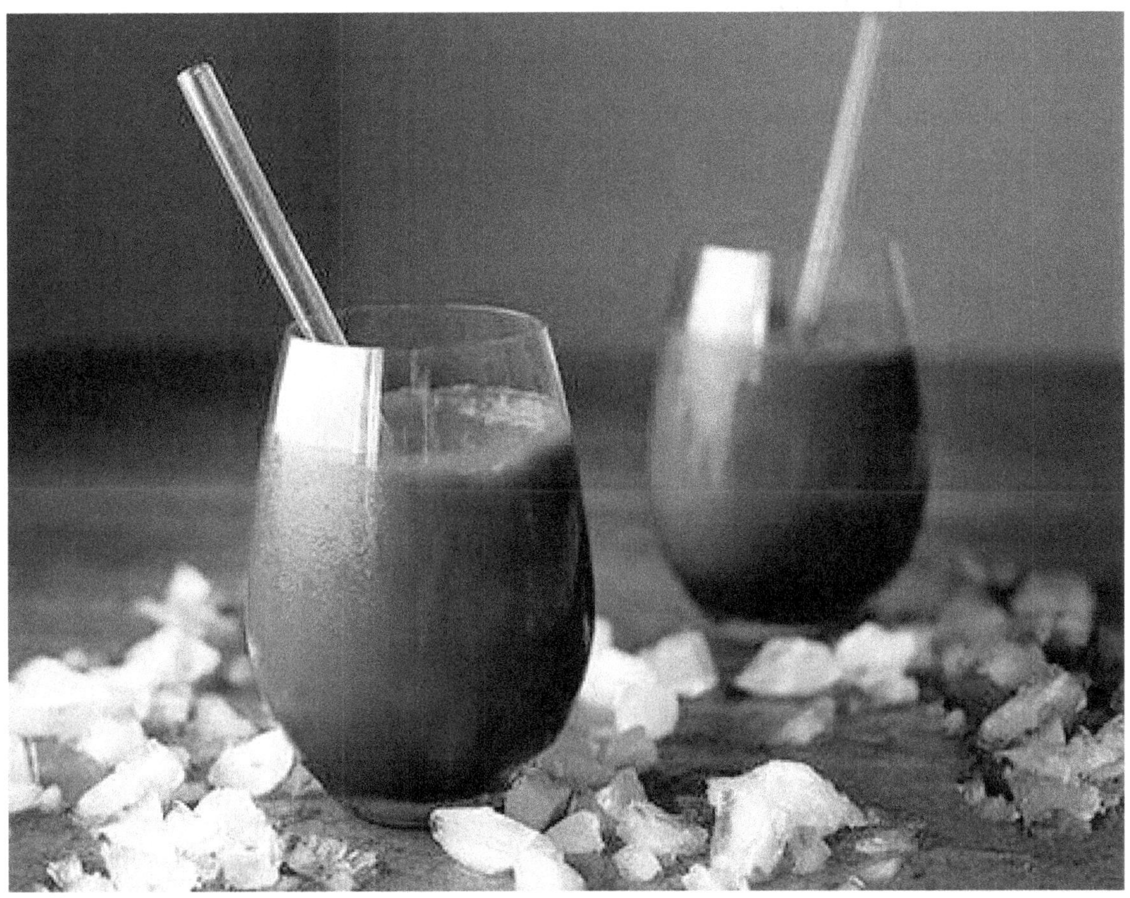

I know people that allow their daughter(s) to drink this juice once a month. The reason being it's packed full of iron, and a growing girl always needs iron. Make sure only use organic ingredients and nothing else.

Makes: 1 glass (10-ounces)

Serving: 1 glass

Ingredients:

- 1 Cup Chilled Coconut Water
- 1 Inch peeled Ginger
- 1 Medium Green Apple
- 1 Medium Beet Cut into Cubes
- 1 Medium Lemon peeled
- Fresh Cilantro to taste

Directions:

First, put all of the ingredients in your blender and blend on high speed for 50 seconds.

TIP:

Use this juice no more than 2 times a week. Beets have a high iron content and you can overdose on your iron intake.

Cucumber-Carrot Detox Juice

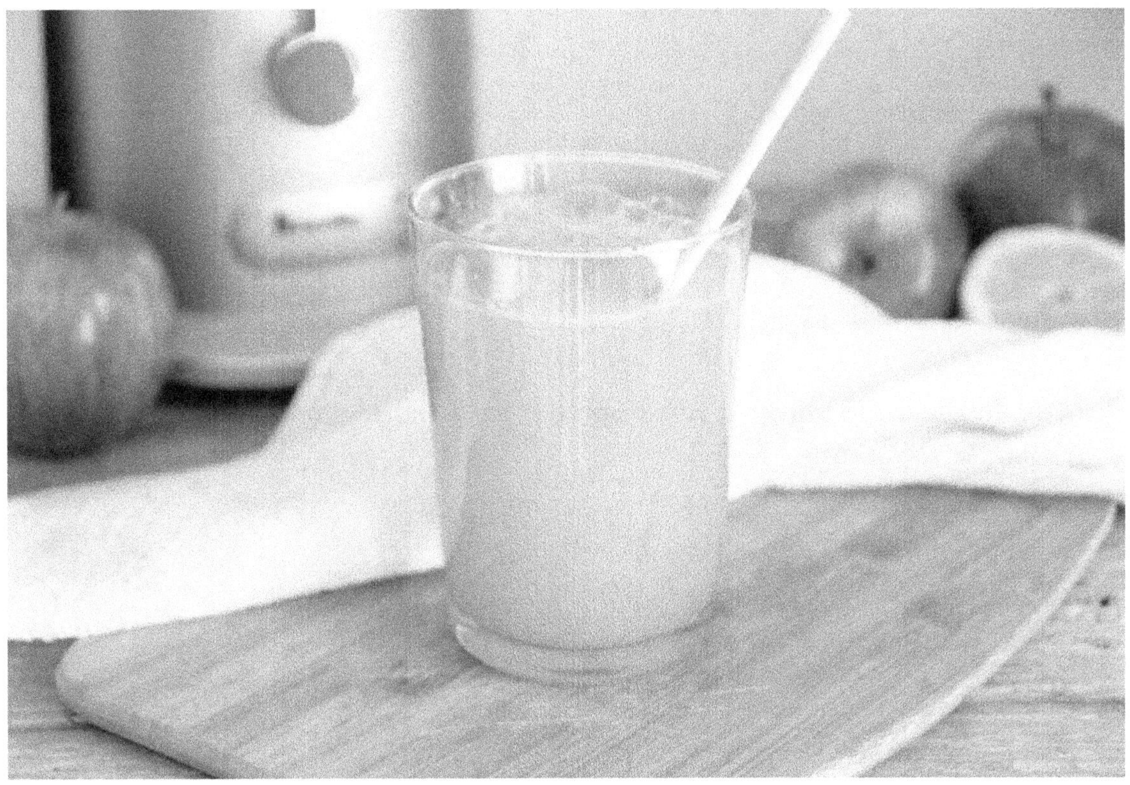

This juice is a lot like the adult version; only this time it's kid-friendly. Ages 8 and up can enjoy this juice.

Makes: 1 cup (8- ounces)

Serving: 1 cup

Ingredients:

- 1 Large peeled Lemon
- 1 Large Cucumber
- 1 Small Beet
- 3 Medium Carrots
- 1 Cup Dandelion Tea (Cooled)

Directions:

Place all the above ingredients in a high-speed blender and 45 seconds or until smooth.

Fill a cup up and enjoy!

Best Green Juice

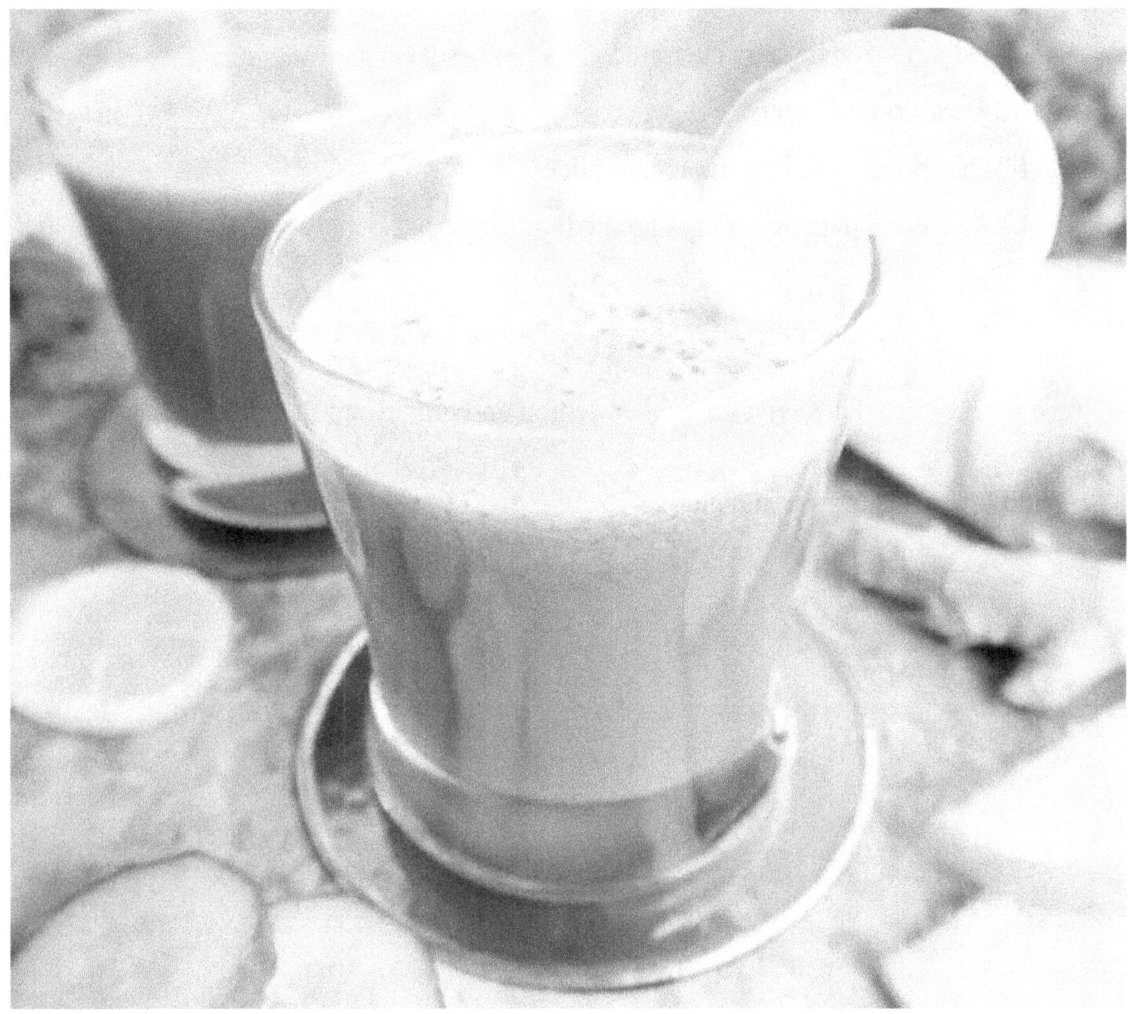

I never knew that starting my day off with fresh fruits and vegetables could make me feel so good!

Makes: 1 glass (8-ounces)

Serving: 1 glass

Ingredients:

- 1 Granny smith apple
- 1 Medium-sized organic cucumber
- 1/2 Pack organic celery
- 1 Tablespoon fresh organic lemon juice
- 1/4 Teaspoon parsley (finely chopped)

Directions:

Using a juicer, juice the celery, cucumber, lemon and granny smith apple.

Then, add in the parsley stir and enjoy.

Cabbage-Blueberry Power Juice

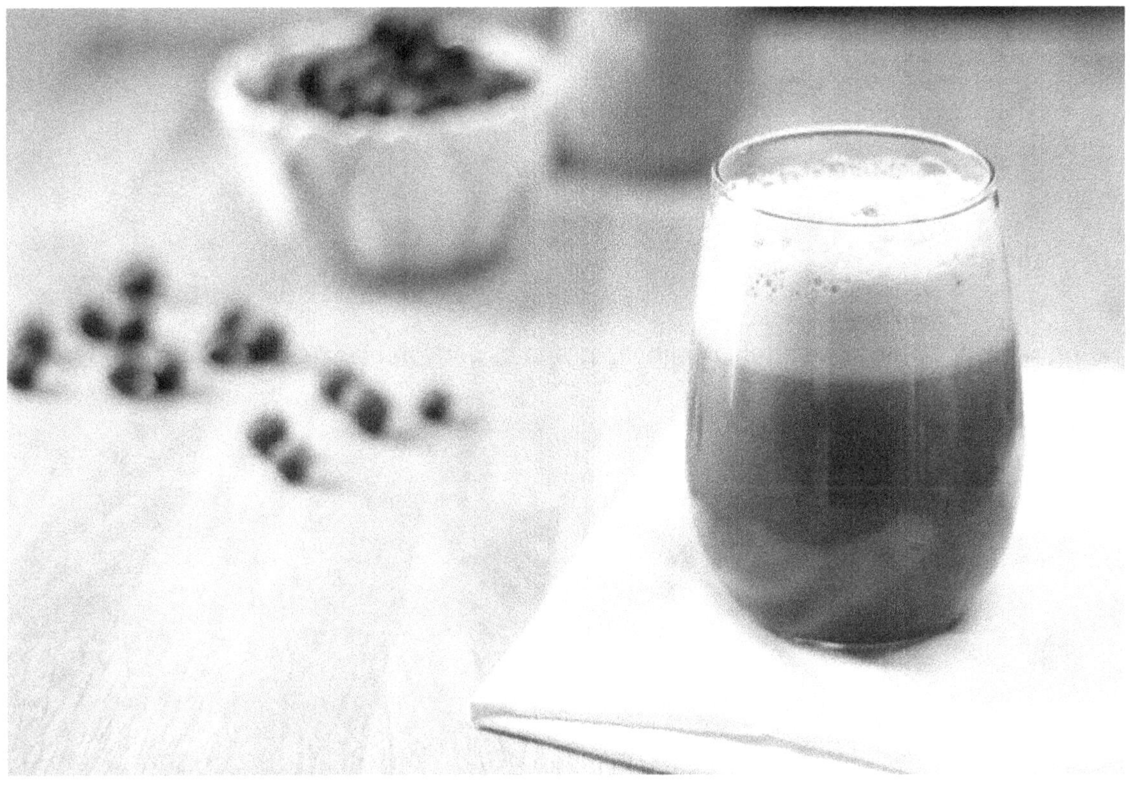

This juice will give you the strength to get started in the mornings without coffee. Trust me, it does work.

Makes: 1 cup (8-ounces)

Serving: 1 cup

Ingredients:

- 1/4 Medium red cabbage
- 1 Large cucumber
- 1 Large apple
- 1 Cup fresh blueberries

Directions:

Using a blender place cucumber, cabbage, apple, and blueberries, into the blender and liquefy

Pour into a glass or water bottle and enjoy.

Apple-Spinach Juice

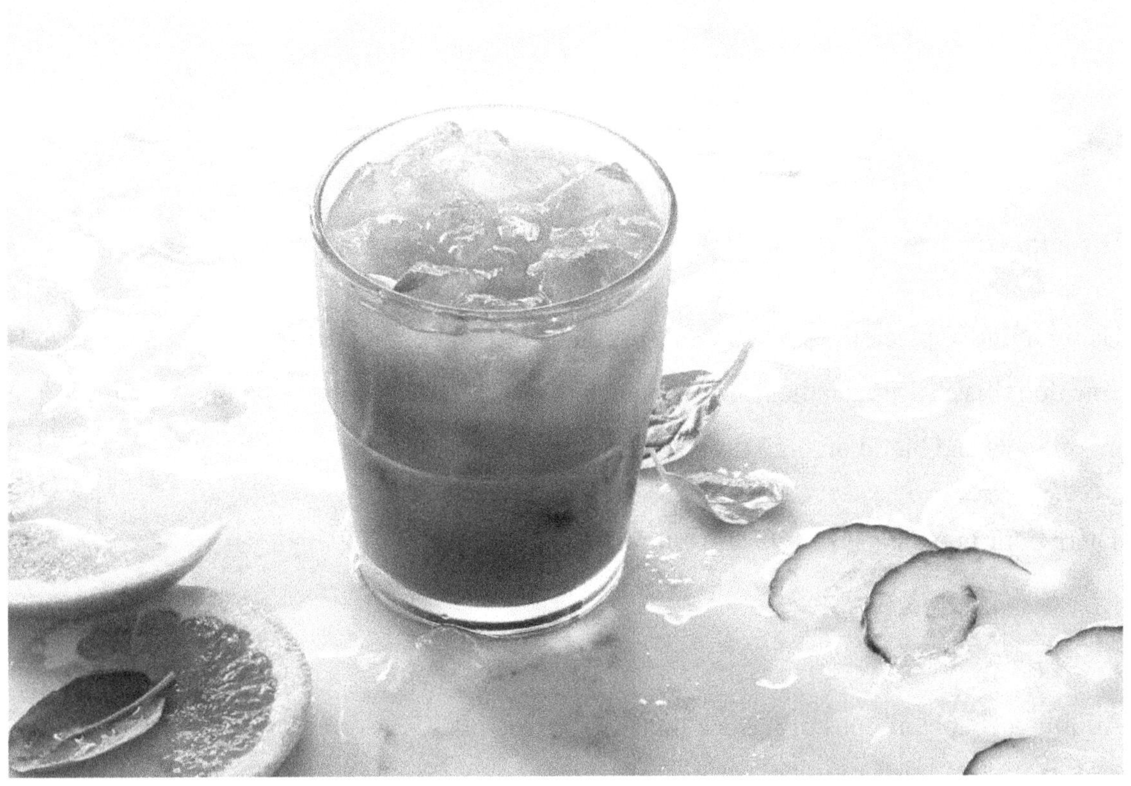

This apple-spinach juice filled with calcium for healthy bones.

Makes: 2 glasses (8-ounces)

Serving size: 1 glass

Ingredients:

- 2 Cups organic spinach
- 1 Large organic grapefruit
- 1 Fresh ginger peeled (1/2 inch)
- 1 Large organic green apple, cut into four's

Directions:

Using a juicer, place the spinach, apple, grapefruit, and ginger into the juicer and juice. If you don't have a juicer then, use a blender. Instead, all you have to do is just add the ingredients and blend on high until smooth.

Then, pour into a glass or two and enjoy!

TIP:

Adding a couple of cubs of ice is a nice treat in the juice.

Orange - Carrot Juice

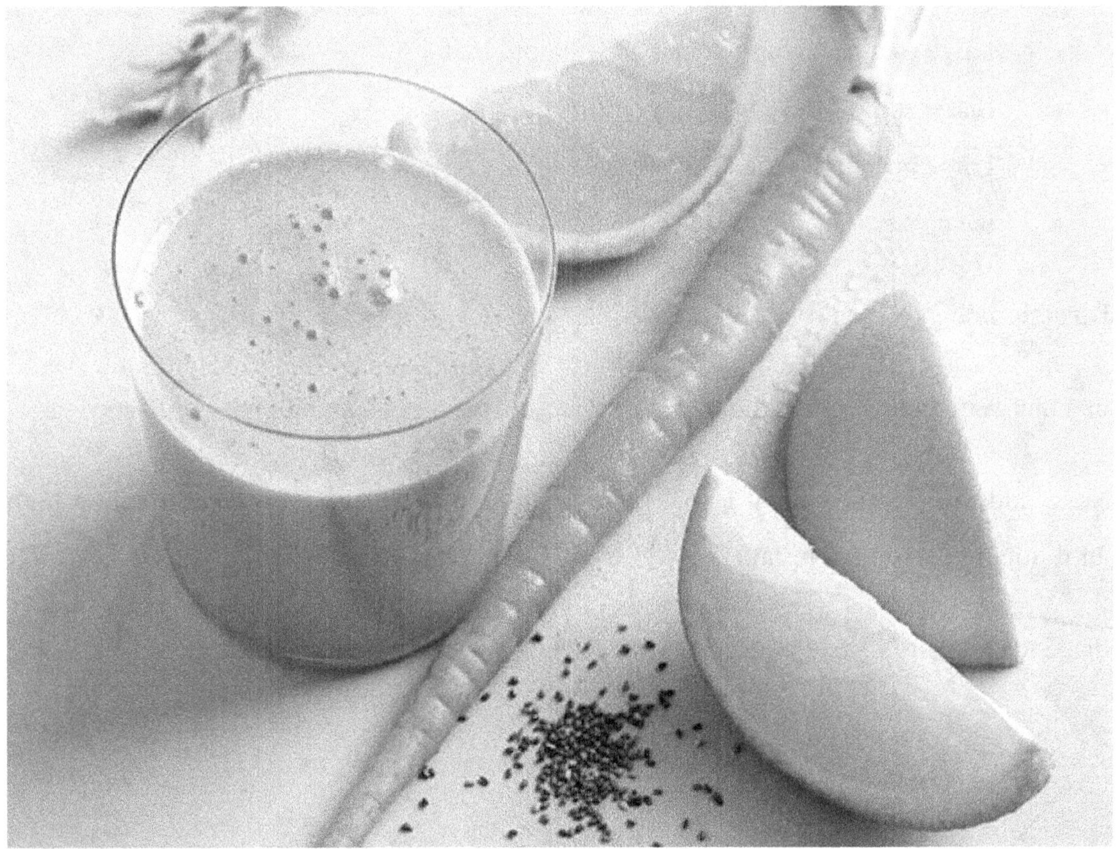

In this energetic, fresh orange carrot detox juice, you'll be adding some extra flavor to everyday orange juice. You will be adding a nice large yellow tomato.

Makes 1 glass (8-ounces)

Serving: 1 glass

Ingredients:

- 1 Large yellow tomato, sliced
- 1 Large orange, skin removed and cut into half
- 1 Large apple
- 4 Large peeled, carrots
- 3 Ice cubes

Directions:

In a blender add the yellow tomato and peeled orange and blend on high for 20 seconds.

Next, add the carrots (one at a time) and apple into the orange mix and blend on high until liquefied. About 1 minute.

Place ice into a glass and pour juice over ice and sip away to good health.

Antioxidant Supreme

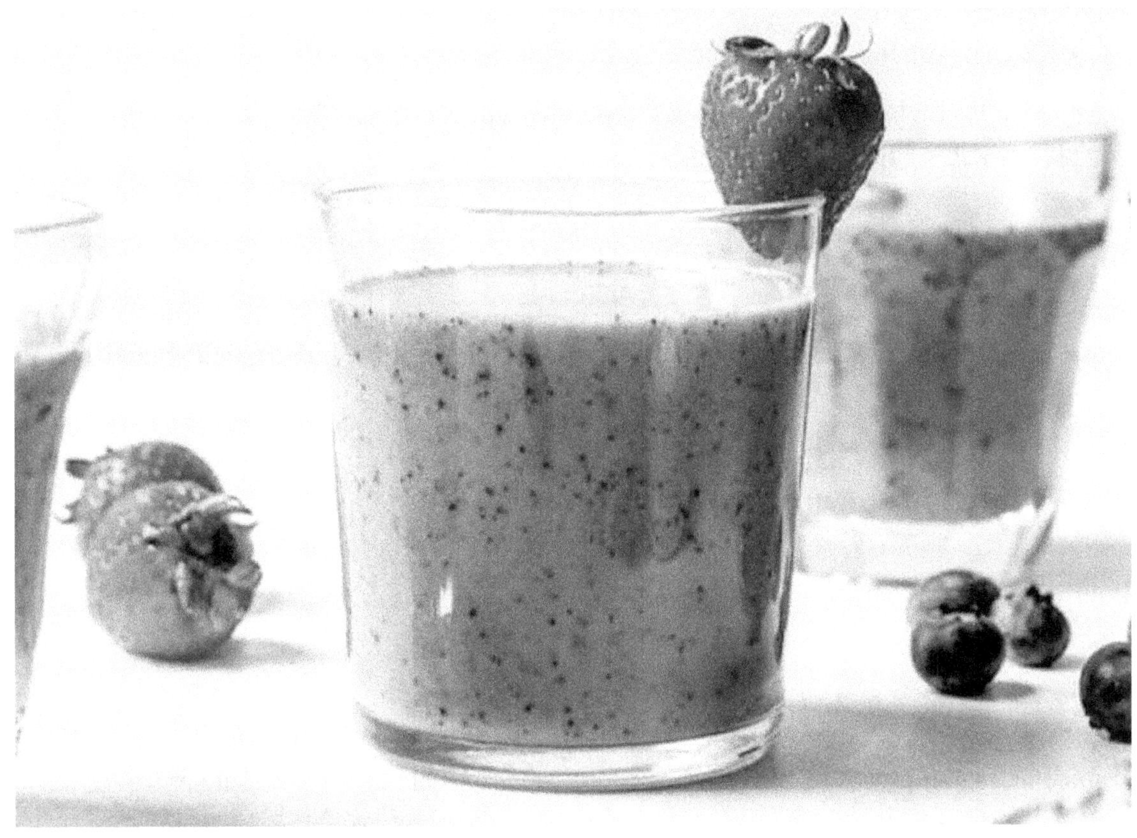

Antioxidants are certainly found in many foods, including berries. They help slow down the aging of the face. In this juice, you will see it has fresh yummy blueberry taste.

Makes 2 cups (8-ounces)

Serving: 1 cup

Ingredients:

- 2 Cups organic blueberries
- 2 Cups organic strawberries
- 3 Cups mango (skin removed and roughly chopped)
- 1/2 Cup cool water

Directions:

Place the water, strawberries, blueberries, and mango, into a blender and blend for 30 seconds.

Scrap down the sides of the cup and blend until juice.

Pour into cups and enjoy

TIP:

If juice has small pieces of the fruit and more water and blend for 1-minute more.

Immune Booster

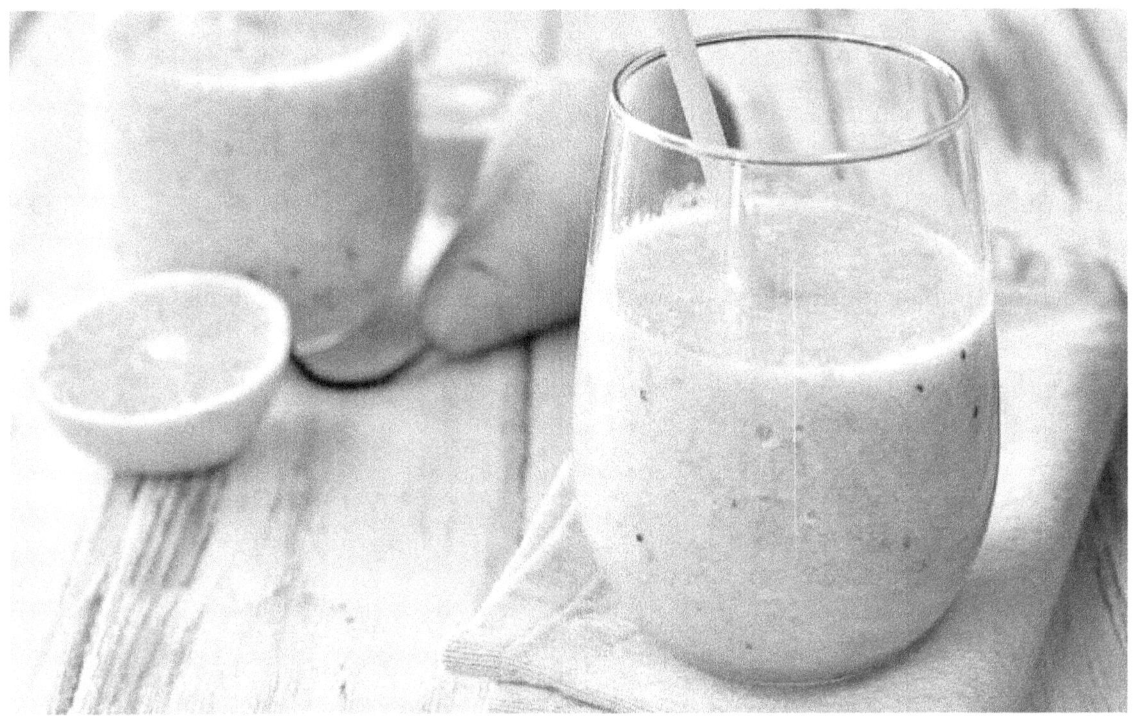

Keep colds away from your family with this detox juice that's packed full of vitamin C.

Makes 2 cups (8-ounces)

Serving: 1 cup

Ingredients:

- 1 Large orange, remove skin and slice into 1/2
- 1 Large grapefruit, remove skin and slice into 1/2
- 3 Kiwis, remove skin and slice into 1/2

Directions:

Into a blender, blend the grapefruit, orange, and kiwis, until smooth and juicy

Pour into a cup and enjoy.

TIP:

It can be stored up to 2 days in your refrigerator.

Fruit-free detox juice

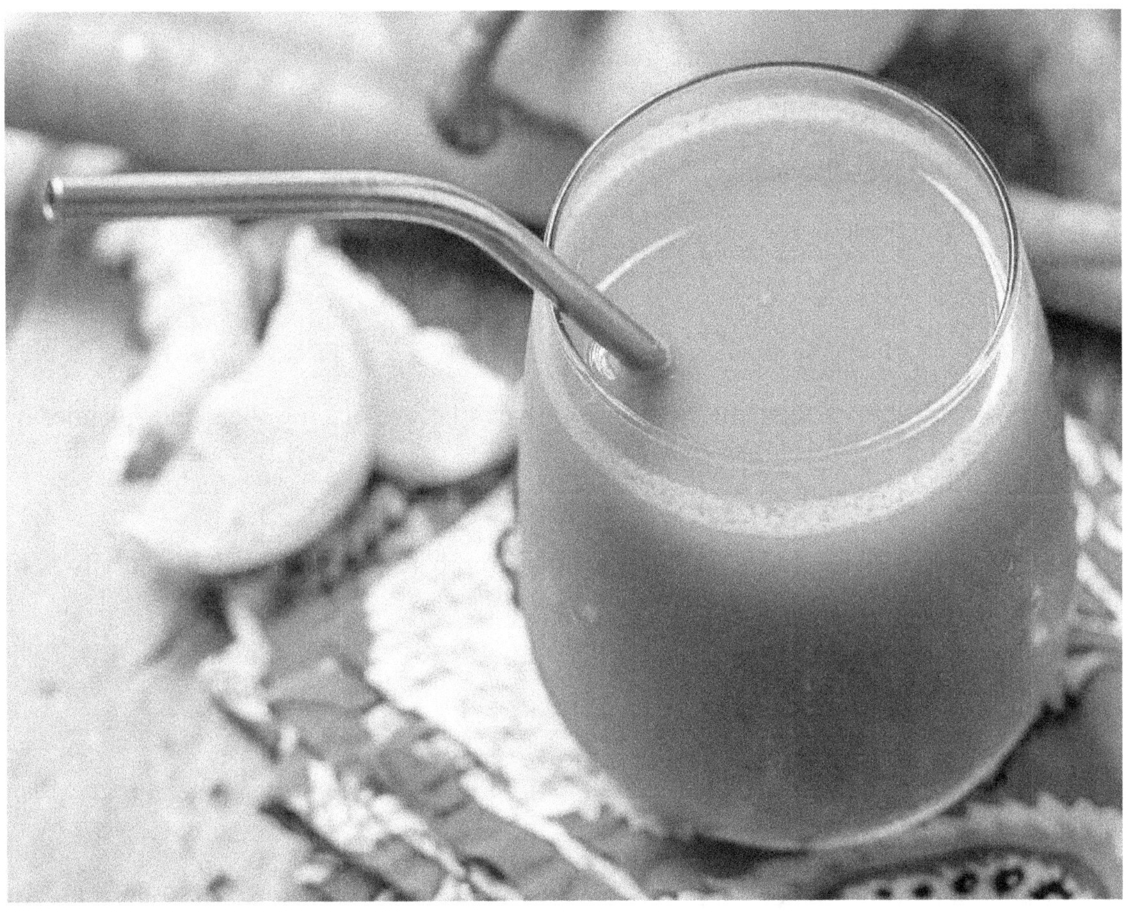

This recipe is great for diabetics because there is no fruit. You will feel good all day with this juice without a sugar high.

Makes: 2 glasses (8-ounces)

Serving: 1 glass

Ingredients:

- 6 Celery stalks
- 6 Carrots remove tops before juicing
- 1 Medium green bell pepper
- 3 Tablespoons flat-leaf parsley
- 1 Lemon, peeled

Directions:

Wash all the vegetables then cut them into quarters before placing them in a blender or juicer.

Using a juicer, push vegetables through shifting from hard to soft. This will actually help to make the juicing easier. See tip for using a blender.

Pour into glasses and drink away.

TIP:

If you are using your blender, add the hard textures a little at a time and blend for 30 seconds. Once they are all blended and the soft vegetables and blend for 1 minute. You might have to work in batches depending on the cup size of the blender.

Glowing Goddess

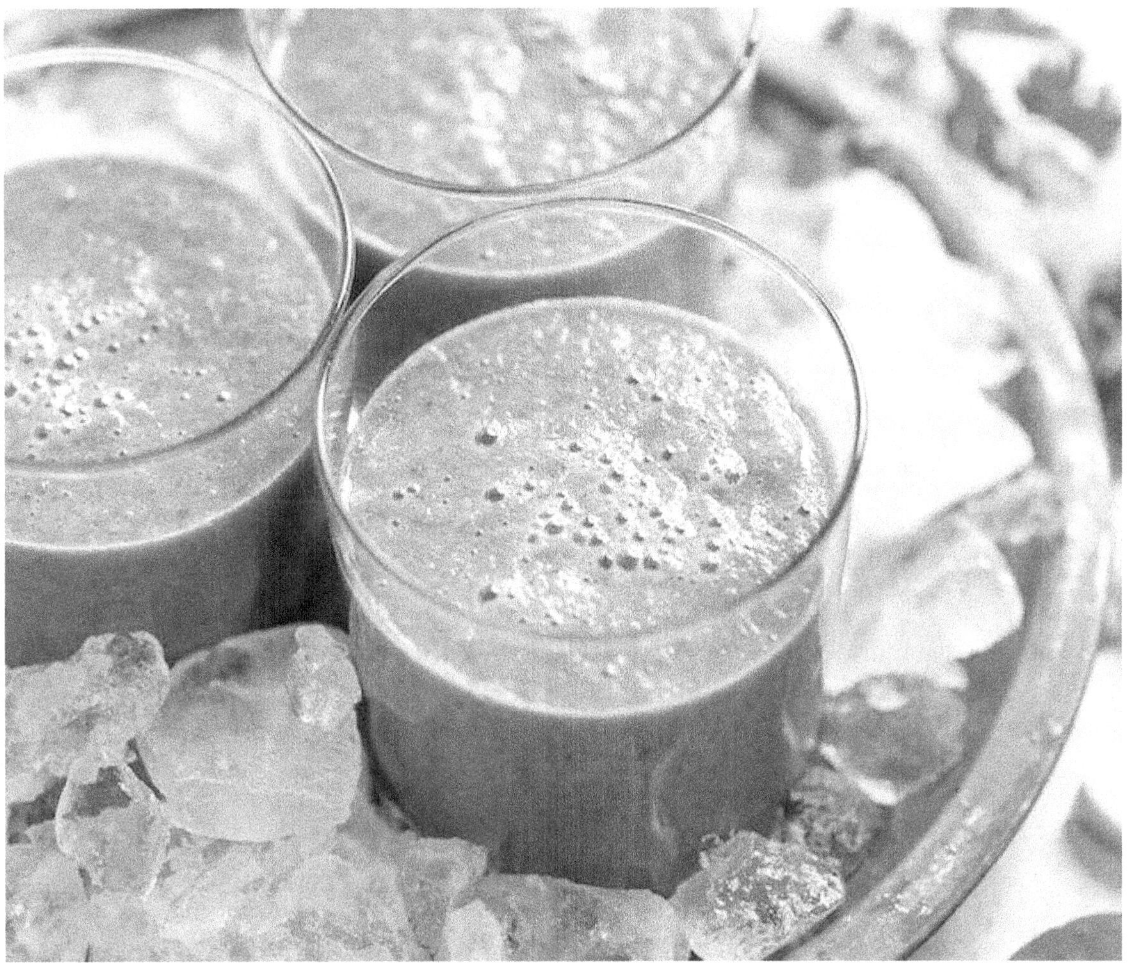

This juice will have your skin looking younger and healthier within days. How? The kale and cilantro are packed full of vitamins that help the blood flow.

Makes: 1 cup (8-ounces)

Serving: 1 cup

Ingredients:

- 1/2 Cup chopped kale
- 5 Celery stalks
- 1 Medium green apple
- 1 Small lemon, seeds removed and peeled
- 1 Medium cucumber
- 1 Tablespoon of cilantro

Directions:

In a blender, place all the hard ingredients first and blend for 30 seconds.

Then, add the soft ingredients and blend until smooth.

Fill your glass and drink away.

Lady in Red

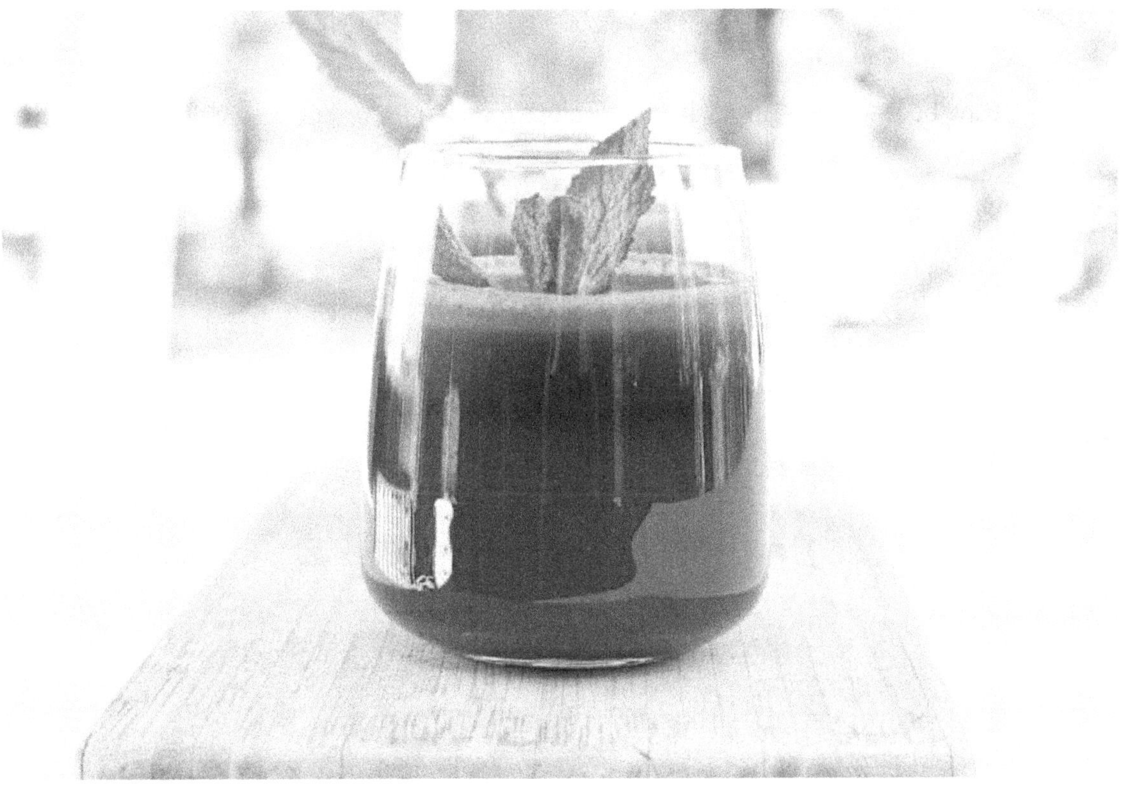

This is a great juice for when you are running low on energy. We all know what the feels like. You only want to rest. No more resting you can, make this drink in the morning and drink at lunch for a great pick up.

Makes: 1 glass (10-ounces)

Serving: 1 glass

Ingredients:

- 2 Medium carrots, washed and peeled
- 1 Medium red apple
- 1 Raw beet washed (use 2 if you don't like beets)

Directions:

In a juicer, add the beets, apple, carrots and, ginger.

Pour into your favorite bottle or glass and stir then drink and enjoy your boost of energy.

Manhattan Beach Sunshine

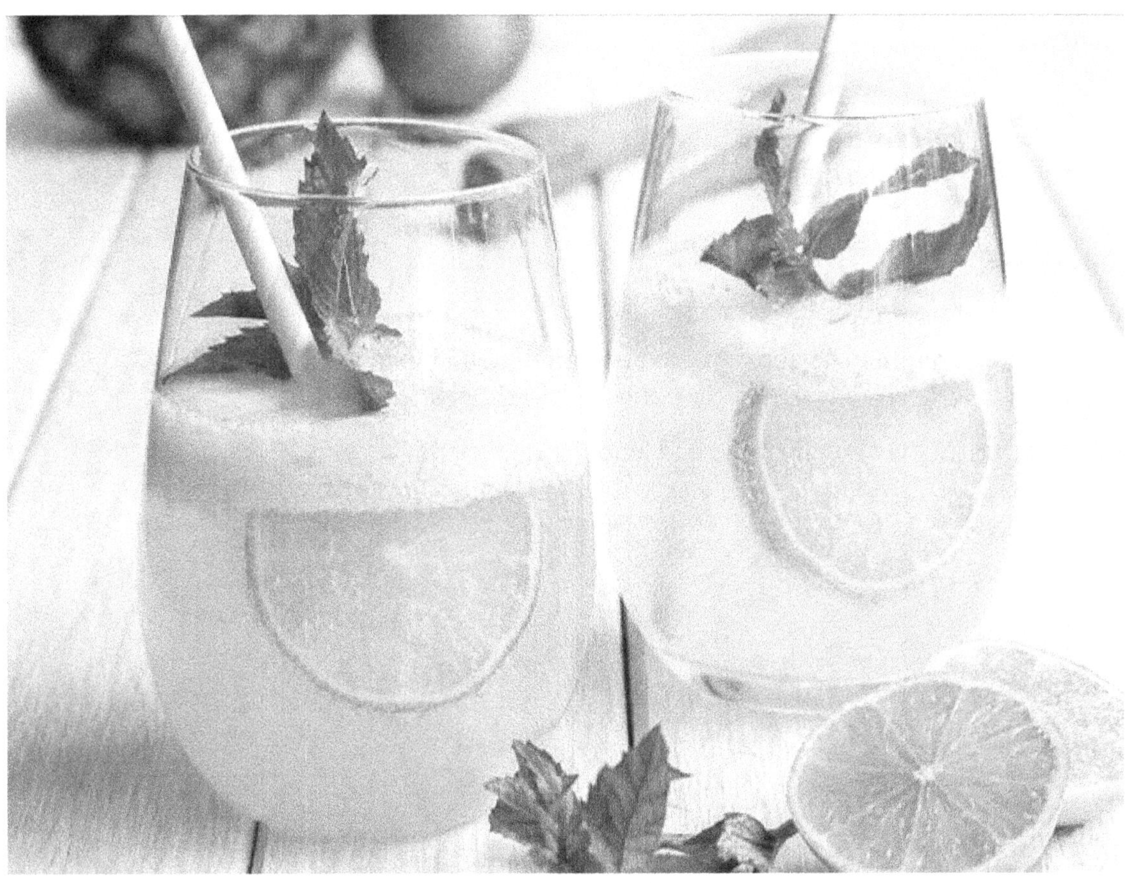

When I am having digestion problems, I drink this juice. It really does help remove the toxins. Also, it's another great juice for immunity!

Makes: 1 glass (8-ounces)

Serving: 1 glass

Ingredients:

- 1 Cup fresh organic pineapple chopped
- 1 Lemon, seeded and peeled
- 1/4 Chopped fresh mint
- 1/4 Piece fresh ginger

Directions:

In a blender, combine the above ingredients firstly and blend until smooth

Fill two glasses evenly with juice and enjoy with a friend.

Anti-aging juice

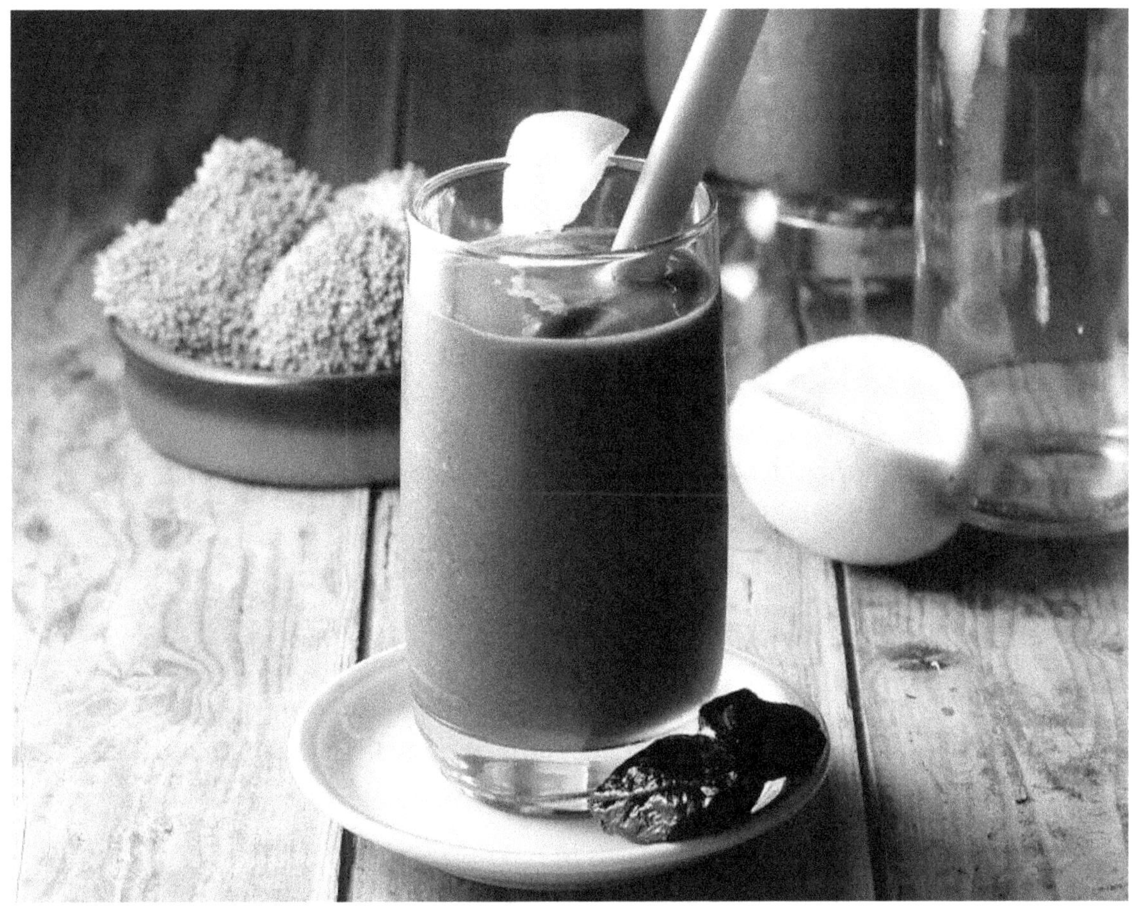

Here is another great juice for looking younger.

Makes 2 cups (8-ounces)

Serving: 1 cup

Ingredients:

- 1 Cup organic fresh blackberries
- 1 Cup organic broccoli
- 1 Small organic cucumber
- 1 Small organic green apple
- 1 Tablespoon watercress
- 4 Teaspoons fresh mint

Directions:

Using a juicer, add the hard textures first and then add the soft ones.

Once all ingredients have been juiced, pour into a glass and enjoy.

TIP:

If drinking alone, put the other serving in the refrigerator until in the morning. Shake well before drinking.

Iron Machine

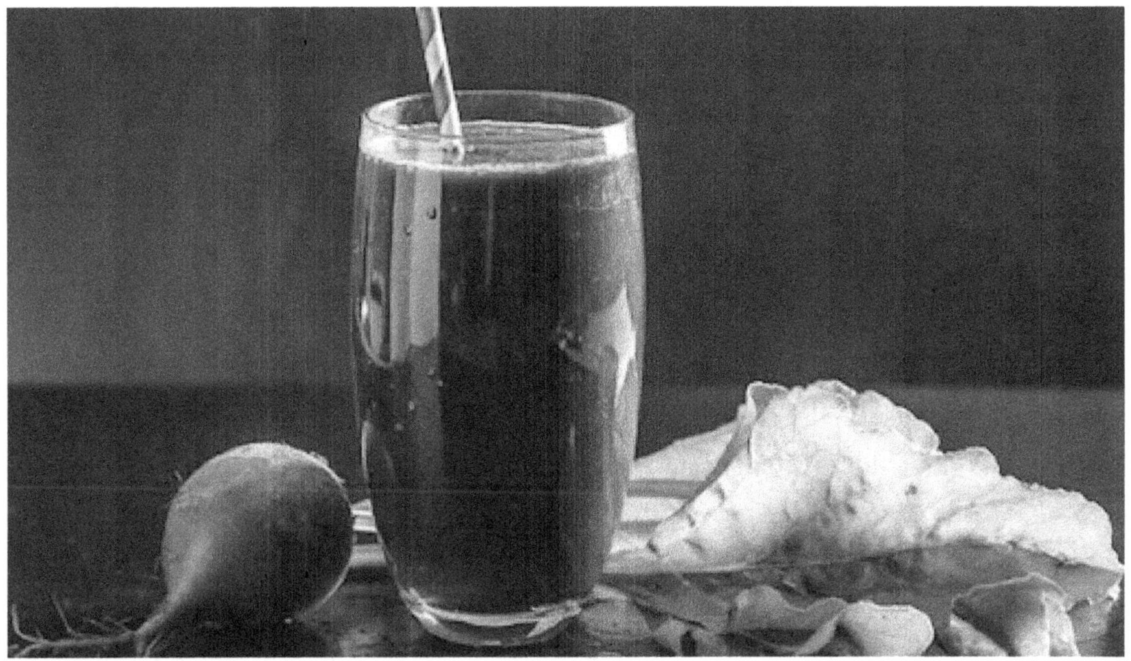

The Iron Machine juice helps to have a healthier complexion. How? Consuming vegetables loaded with carotenoids, like spinach and carrots. These vegetables will truly add light to the surface of your skin.

Makes 2 glasses (8-ounces)

Serving: 1 glass

Ingredients:

- 1 Beet, peeled and divided
- 6 Carrots washed (remove tops)
- 1 Celery stalk
- 1/4 Cup parsley (loosely packed)
- 1 Cup spinach (loosely packed)

Directions:

Using a juicer, add the vegetables one at a time as listed above. You can check the manufactures directions just to be sure how to juice.

Fill a glass or two and drink with a loved one.

Liver detox juice

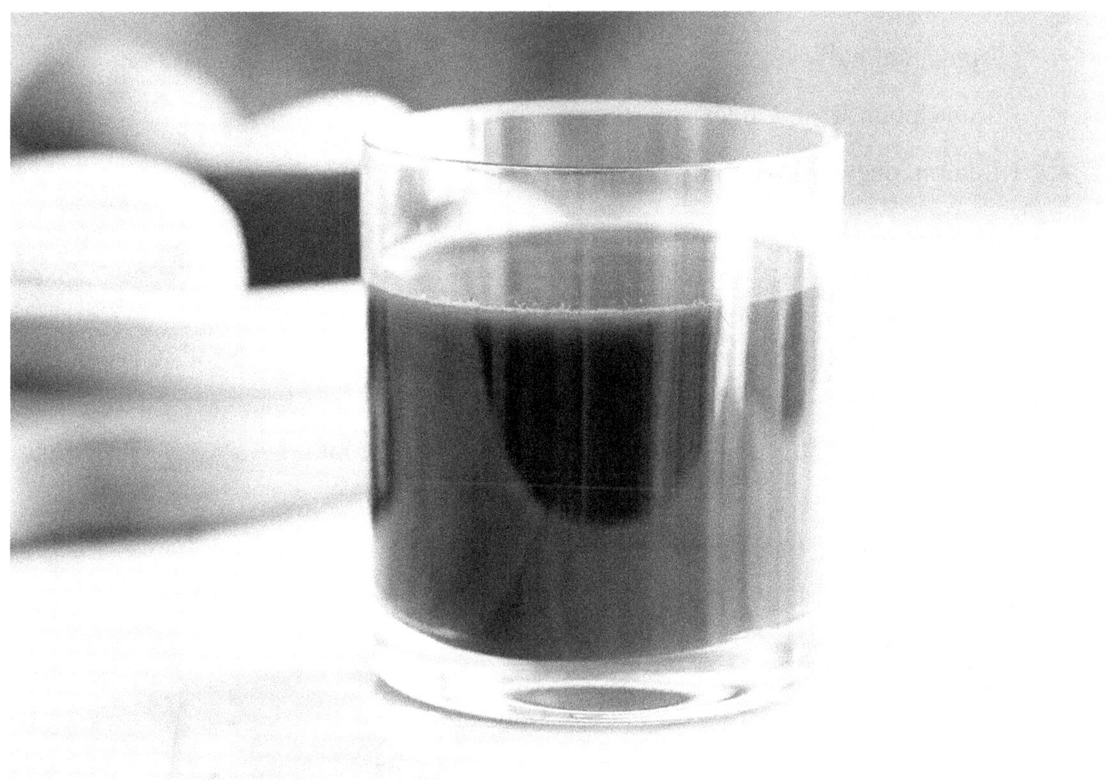

This juice will kick start your liver.

Makes: 1 cup (8-ounces)

Serving: 1 cup

Ingredients:

- 1 Beet, divided cut in half
- 1 Apple, cut half
- 1 Tablespoon fresh ginger
- 1 Lemon, peel removed

Directions:

Using a blender, place the beet and apple into the cup and blend on high for 30 seconds.

Add remaining ingredients and blend for a minute or until smooth.

Fill up a glass and drink away to a better liver.

Clear skin juice

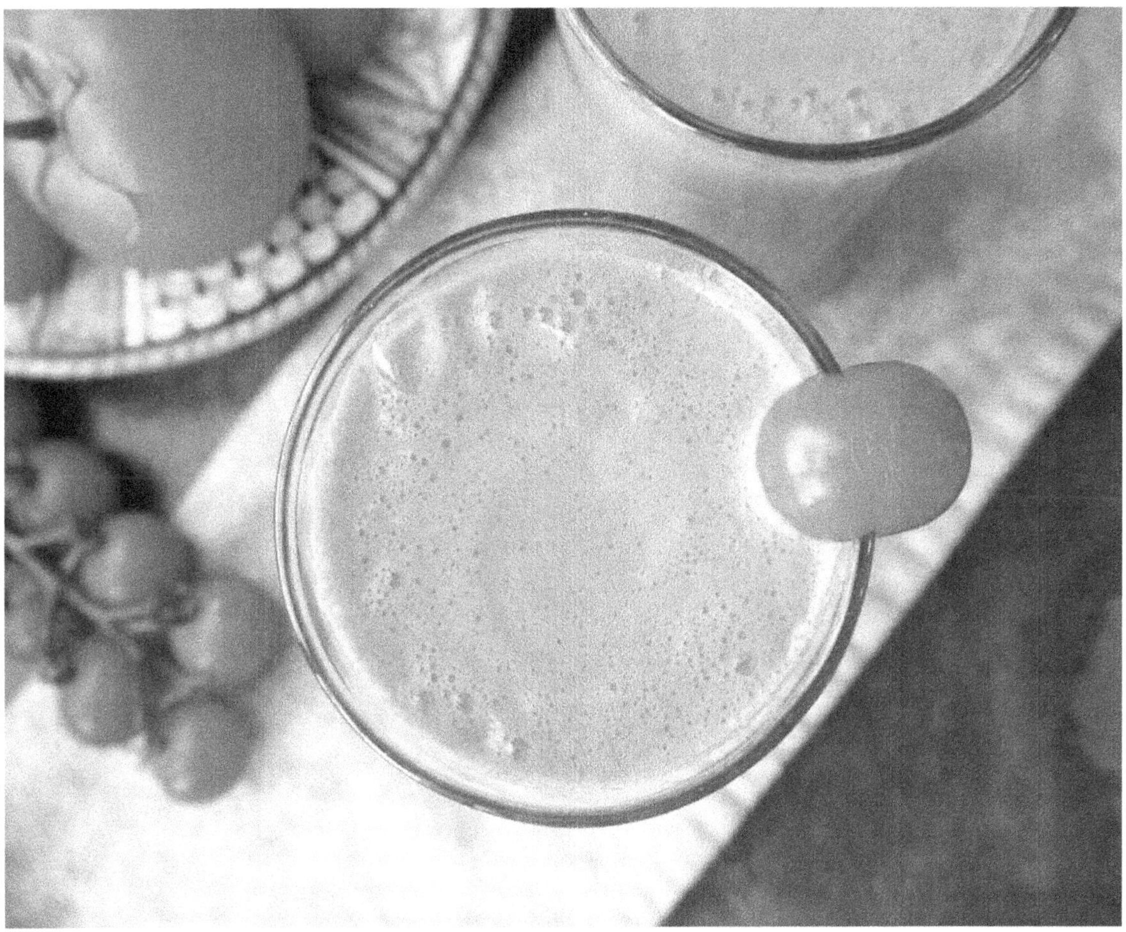

The Clear Skin Juice packed full of phosphorous and potassium. Both help reduce stress. Stress can cause acne. This juice will help with acne and stress.

Makes 2 cups (8-ounces)

Serving: 1 cup

Ingredients:

- 1 Cup fresh blueberries
- 1 Medium granny smith apple
- 1 Medium organic tomato
- 1 Broccoli stalk chopped
- 6 Large carrots washed and peeled

Directions:

First, place the above ingredients in a blender and blend for 1 minute or until smooth.

Fill a cup and enjoy!

Kale Whale

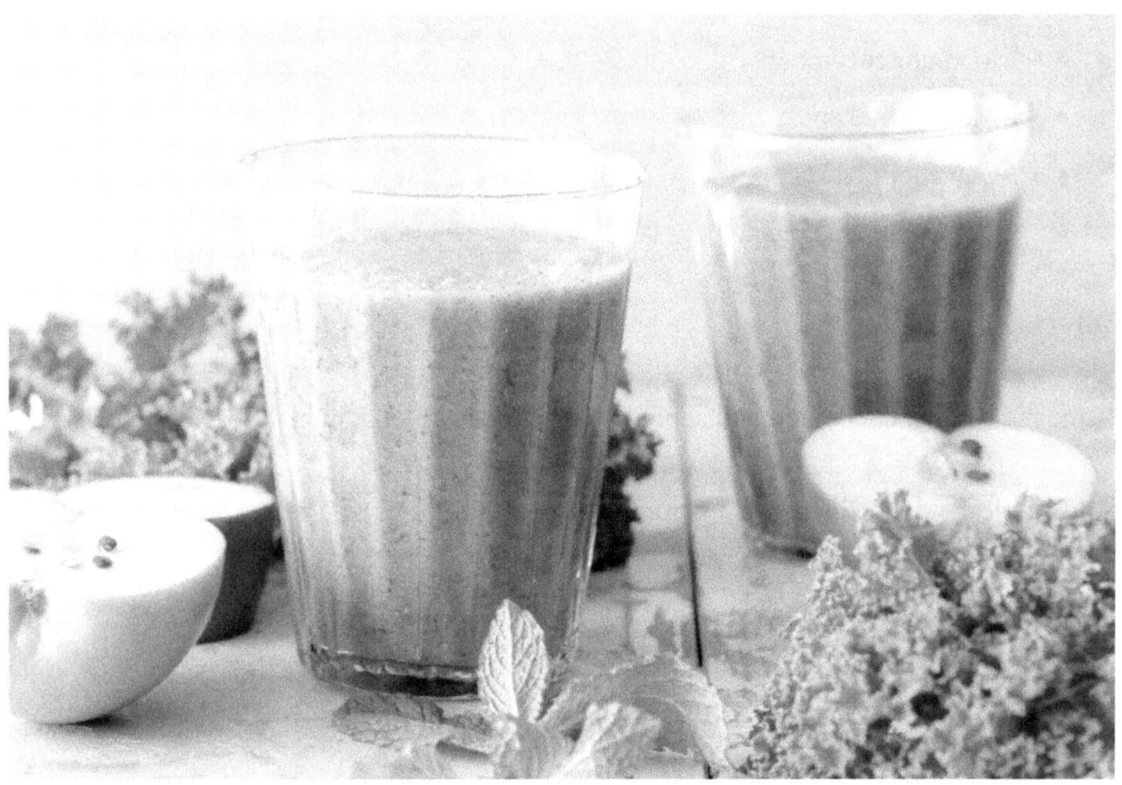

Do you want a better way to battle acne? Then, try Kale Whale Juice. It's loaded with helpful nutrients, like minerals and vitamins. Within a few days of drinking this juice, you will start to see a change.

Makes: 1 cup (8-ounces)

Serving: 1 cup

Ingredients:

- 3 Carrots
- 1 Medium cucumber
- 1 Medium red apple
- 1 Cup chopped kale
- 1/2 Cup chopped parsley

Directions:

Place the carrots, cucumber, and apple in a blender and blend on high for 35 seconds.

Add parsley and kale blend on high until smooth.

Pour into a glass and drink acne away.

Lemon, Cucumber, and Kale Juice

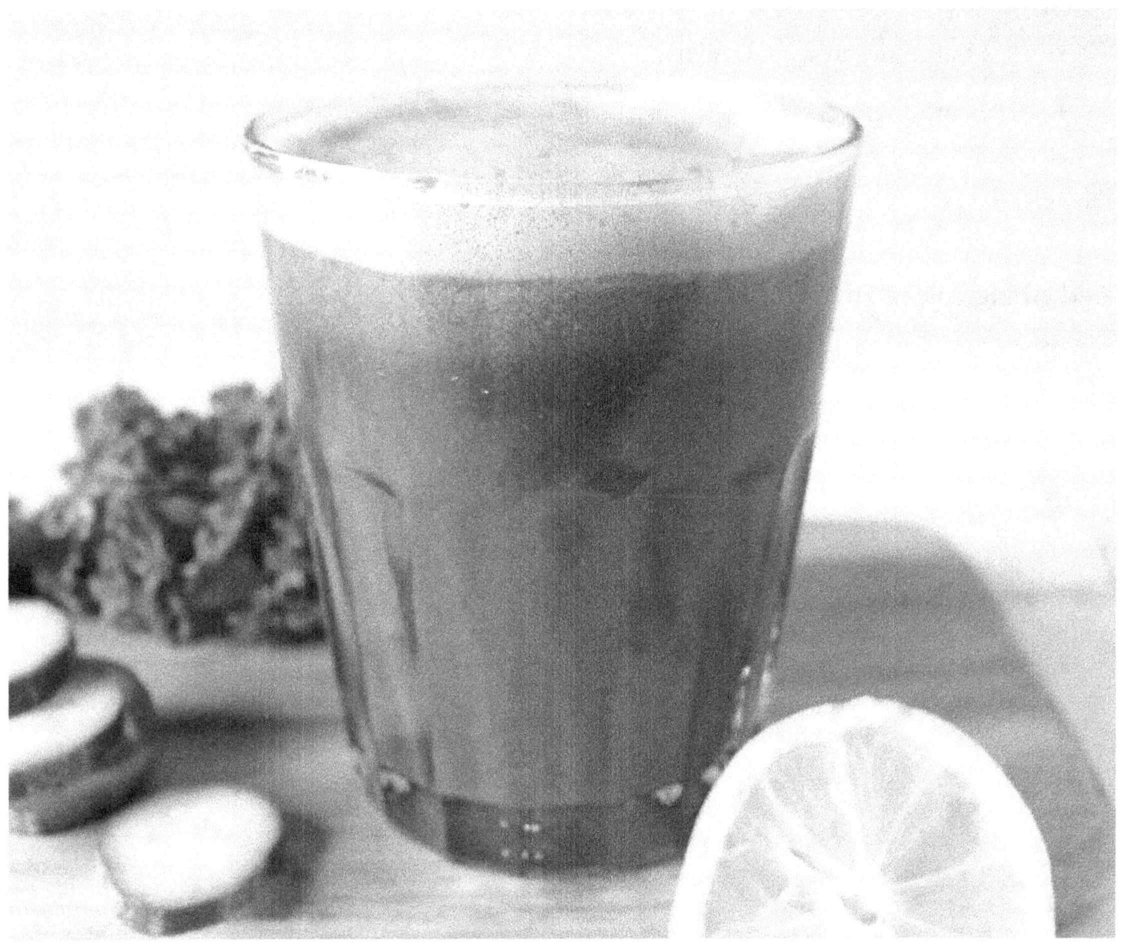

This juice is a lot like the Kale Whale recipe. However, lemon is added to give you vitamin C. Vitamin C benefits the skin. It **Makes** the skin brighter and it removes toxins. Acne feeds of toxins in the body.

Makes: 1 glass (8-ounces)

Serving: 1 glass

Ingredients:

- 4 Large organic kale stalks
- 1/2 Large organic cucumber
- 1/2 Large lemon

Directions:

Add all ingredients into a blender, then blend until smooth.

Pour into a glass.

Kiwi Juice

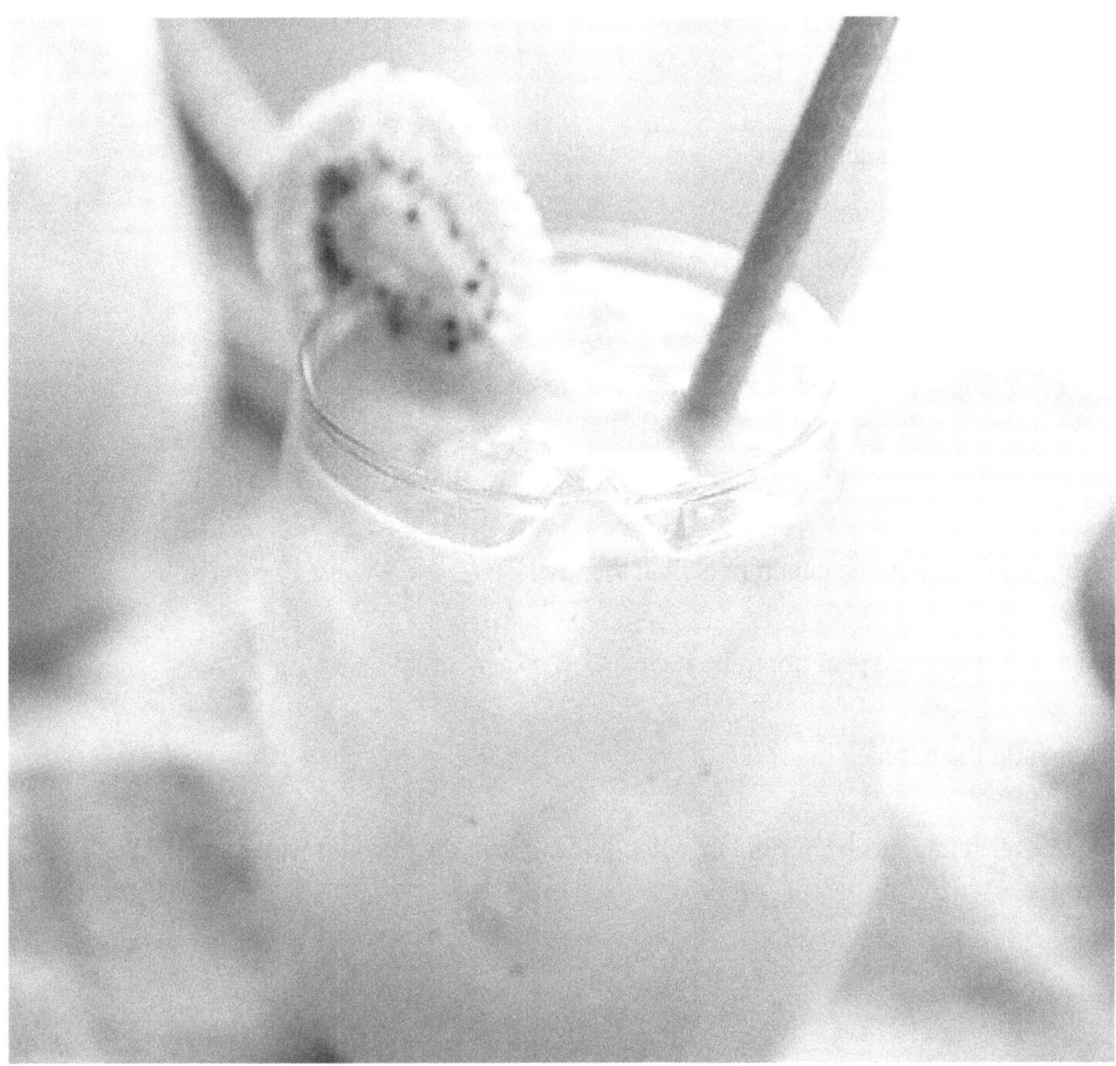

Kiwis are loaded with vitamin C. Vitamin C works as an antioxidant in our bodies. It not only helps to fight colds, it's also great in fighting acne. Why? Because of being an anti-inflammatory as well.

Makes: 1 cup (8-ounces)

Serving: 1 cup

Ingredients:

- 3 Large kiwis
- 3 Medium cucumbers
- 2 Medium limes
- 1 Small pear
- 1 Cup organic coconut water
- 1 Cup baby cos lettuce/romaine lettuce chopped

Directions:

Using a juicer, add the cucumbers than the kiwis.

Next, the limes and pear are to be juiced.

Then, add the lettuce.

Once everything has been run throw the juicer stir in the coconut water and drink.

Watermelon Juice

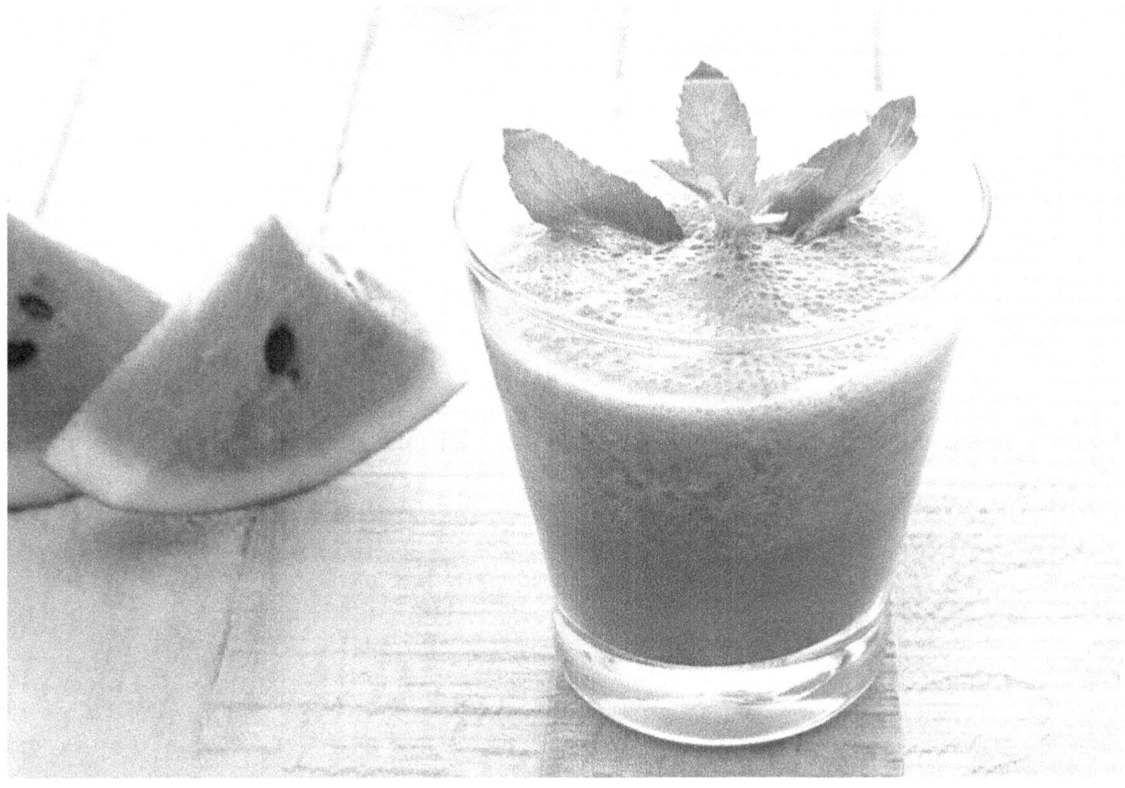

Watermelon can help with blood sugars and skin. The trick is only to use the natural sugar found in the watermelon and not add more.

Makes: 1 glass (8-ounces)

Serving: 1 glass

Ingredients:

- 2 Cups watermelon (fruit only)
- 1/4 Cup chopped mint leaves
- 1/4 Teaspoon lime juice

Directions:

Place 1 cup watermelon in a blender and blend on high for 1 minute. Pour into a small jar and repeat with remaining watermelon.

Place 3 tablespoons of the juice back into the blender and add the mint and lime juice. Blend for 30 seconds.

Now, pour this mixture into the jar with the juice and stir.

Drink and enjoy.

Carrot-Apple Glow Juice

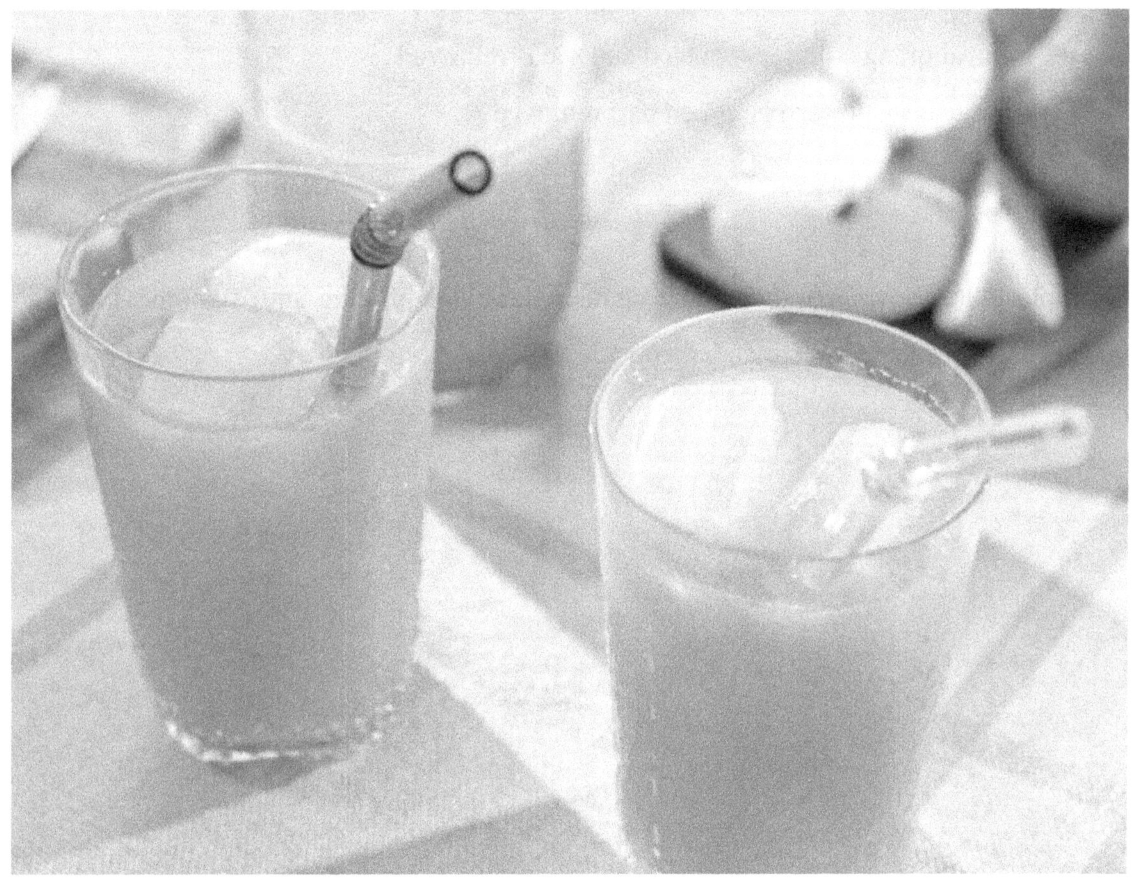

Did you know carrots are high in vitamin A.? Even though vitamin A supports better eyesight, it can also fight acne and many different skin problems. Carrot juice is also a great detox juice.

Makes 1 cup (8-ounces)

Serving: 1 cup

Ingredients:

- 1 Large organic Granny Smith apple, chopped
- 1 Naval orange, divided, peeled and seeds removed
- 2 Large organic carrots, green part removed

Directions:

First, place the above ingredients in a blender and blend on high until smooth. If need to add a little tap water for the blender to work well.

Sweet Potato Juice

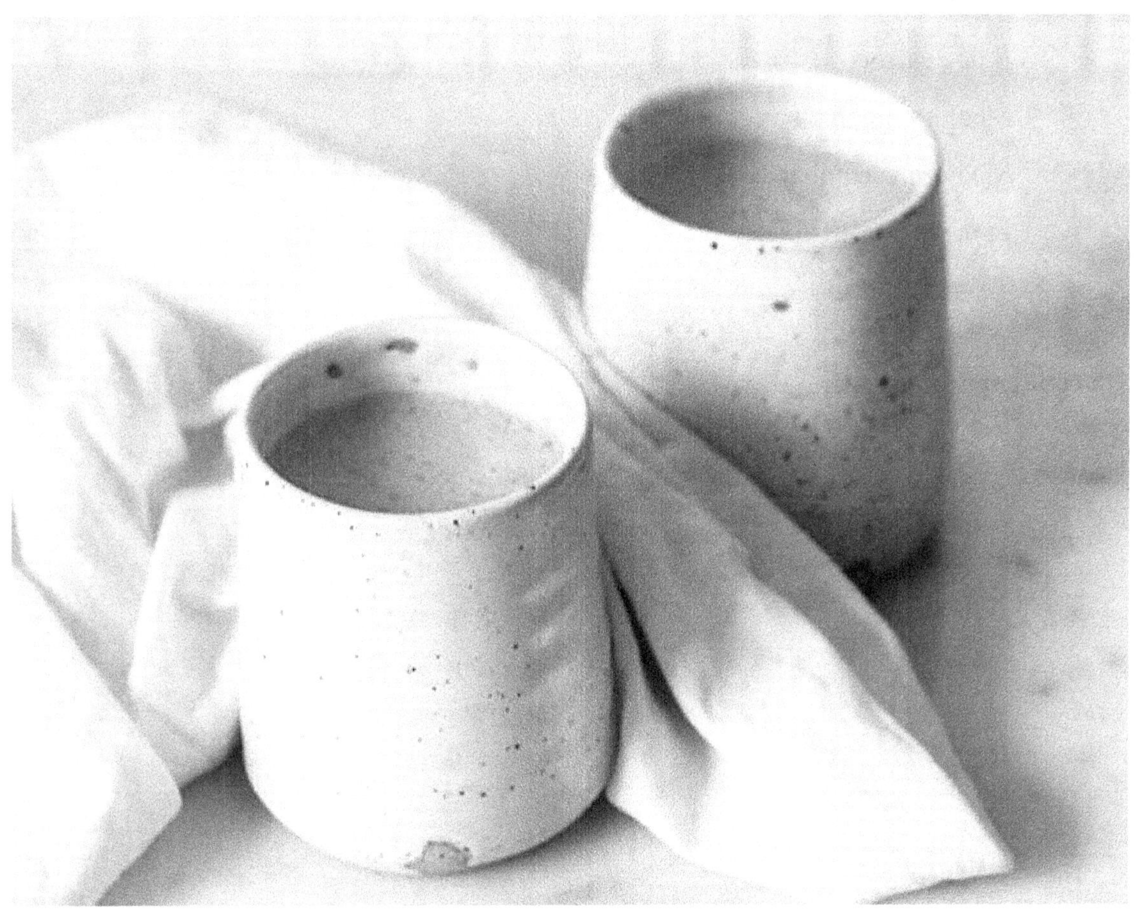

Sweet potato juice is another acne fighting drink to try.

Makes: 1 cup (8-ounces)

Serving: 1 cup

Ingredients:

- 4 Celery stalks
- 3 Large carrots
- 1 Medium organic sweet potato
- 1 Medium cucumber
- 1 Lemon
- 2 Teaspoon turmeric root powder

Directions:

Using a blender, add the vegetables and blend until smooth

Pour into a cup and enjoy.

Green Juice to Help Lower Blood Pressure

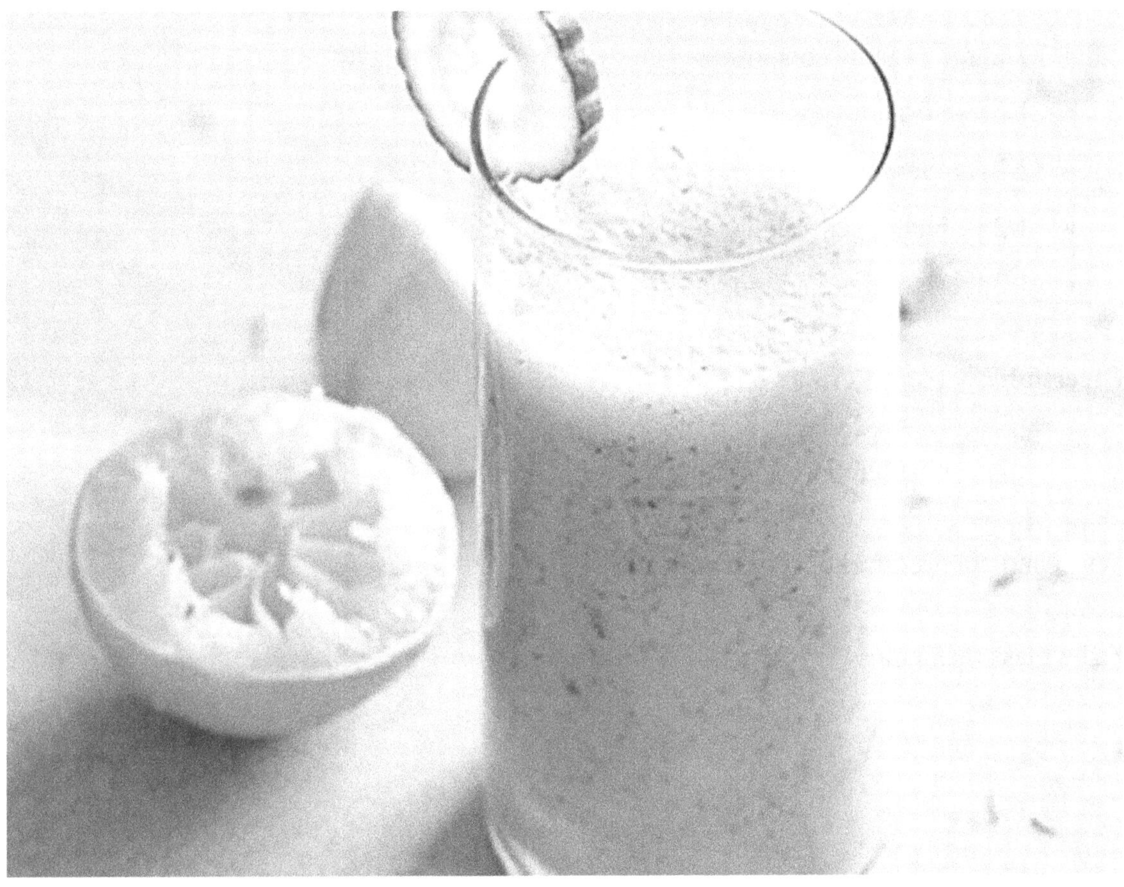

Drinking this juice will help you to maintain good blood pressure.

Makes: 1 glass (10-ounces)

Serving: 1 glass

Ingredients:

- 4 Organic celery sticks
- 2 Large organic cucumbers
- 1 Fresh organic green apple
- 1 Large lemon
- 1/2 Cup chopped parsley
- 1 Tablespoon grated ginger

Directions:

Wash and peel the lemon.

Wash and cut produce to fit into your juicer.

Fill a glass then enjoy!

An Alkalizing Juice

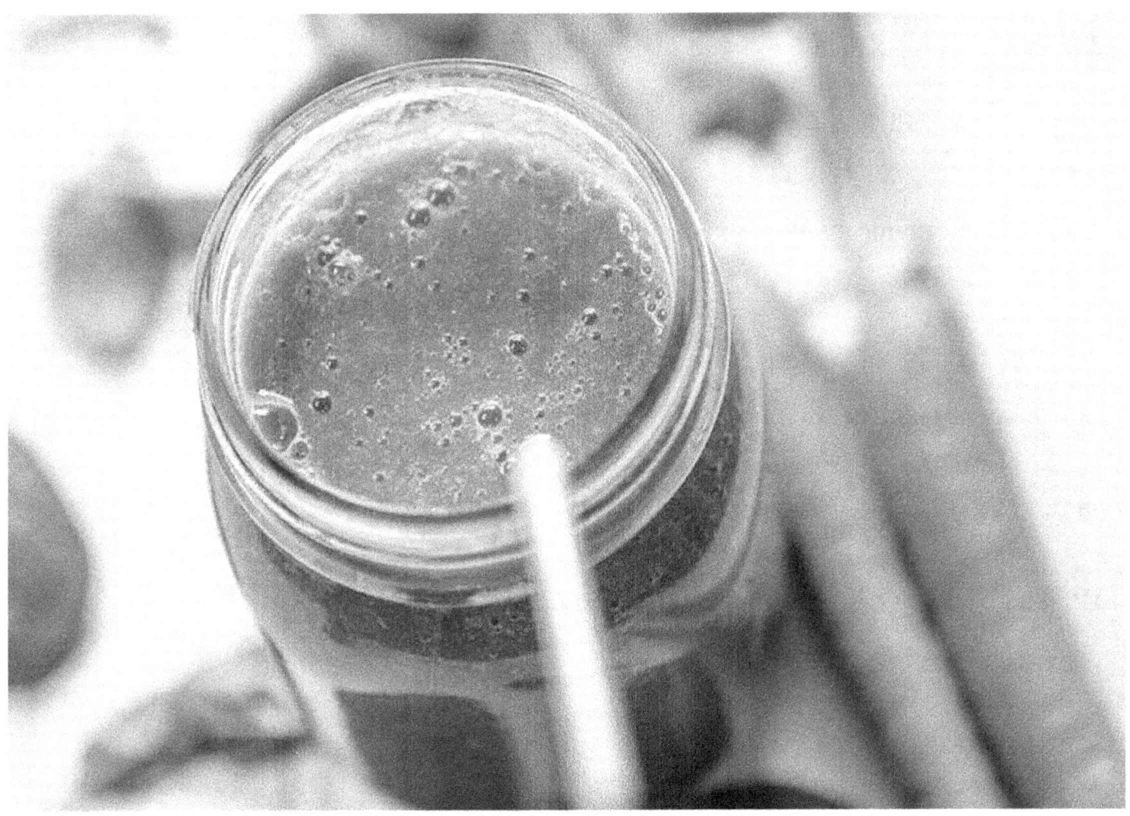

Alkalinity is important for your bodies to be healthy. The cells within our bodies require a natural balance of alkalinity. This will keep your cells and other body parts in good health.

Makes:1 glass (8-ounces)

Serving: 1 glass

Ingredients:

- 1 Organic carrot
- 1 Large cucumber
- 1 Green apple
- 5 Organic celery stalks
- 1 Cup organic spinach

Directions:

Place the carrot, apple, and celery first into a juicer, then add the cucumber and spinach.

Pour and serve.

TIP: To help keep a lower blood sugar level omit carrot.

A Twisted Veggie Juice

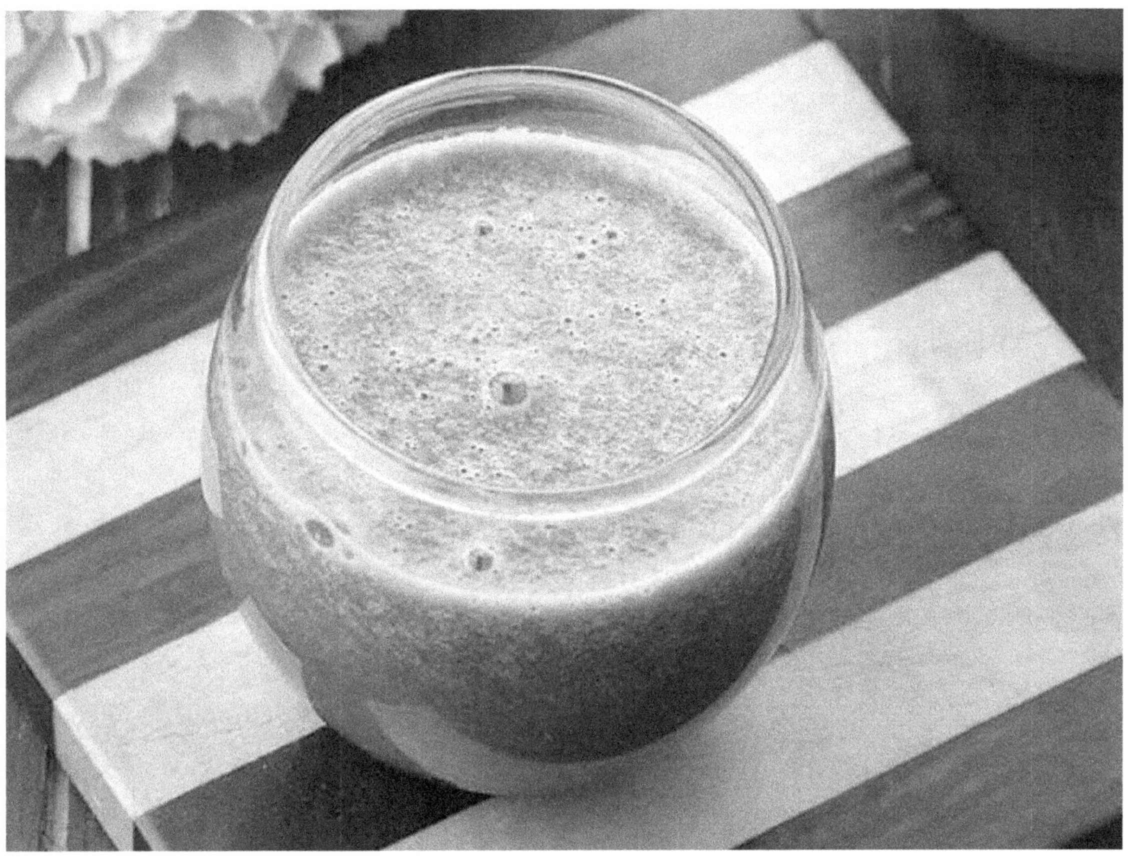

Veggies with lime are really good. So, when I saw the recipe, I know it would be good. I like the idea of it being diabetic safe.

Makes: 1 cup (8-ounces)

Serving: 1 cup

Ingredients:

- 1 Lime
- 1 Medium red pepper
- 1 Small carrot
- 1 Small cucumber
- 1/4 Fennel
- 1/4 Cup cilantro
- 1 Cup chopped spinach

Directions:

First, add all the above ingredients into a blender and blend until smooth.

Pour into a glass and squeeze the lime juice into the juice.

An Energizing Juice

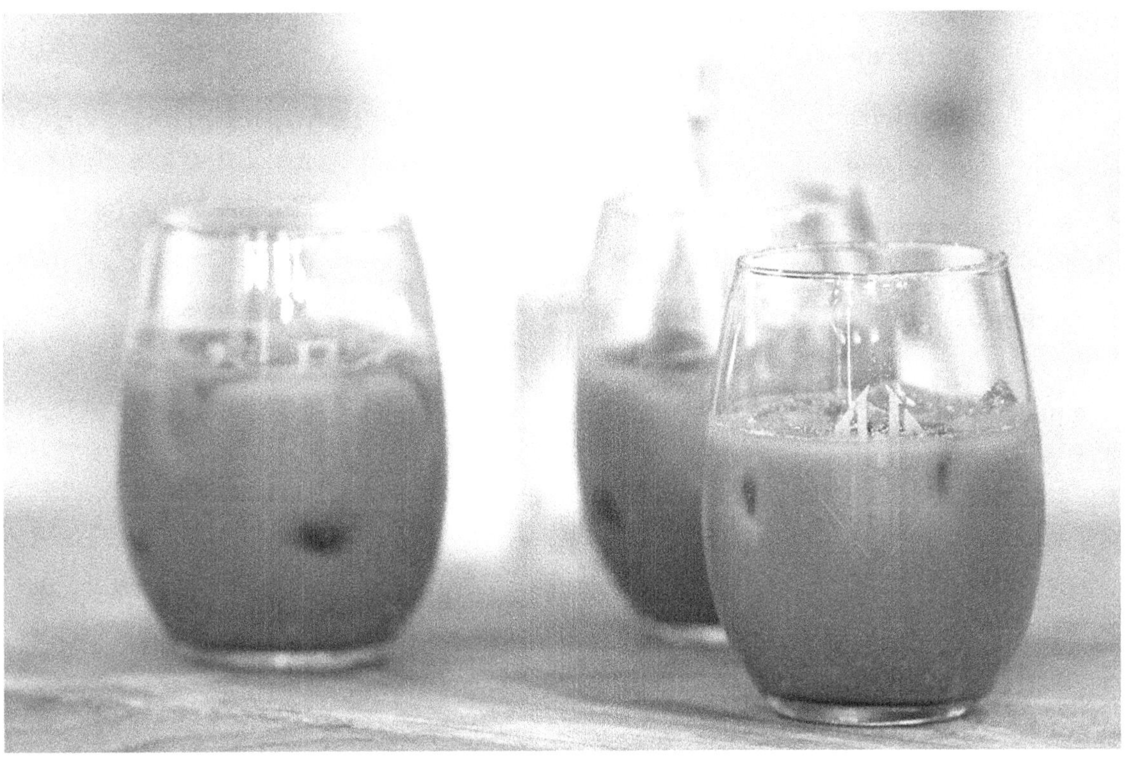

The kale and spinach will give you a power boost.

Makes: 1 glass (8-ounces)

Serving: 1 glass

Ingredients:

- 6 Leaves kale
- 1 Large cucumber
- 5 Celery stalks
- 2 Cups spinach
- 1 Tablespoons parsley

Directions:

In a juicer, place the hard veggies first, then add the soft ones

Once juiced, serve.

B6 Bounty

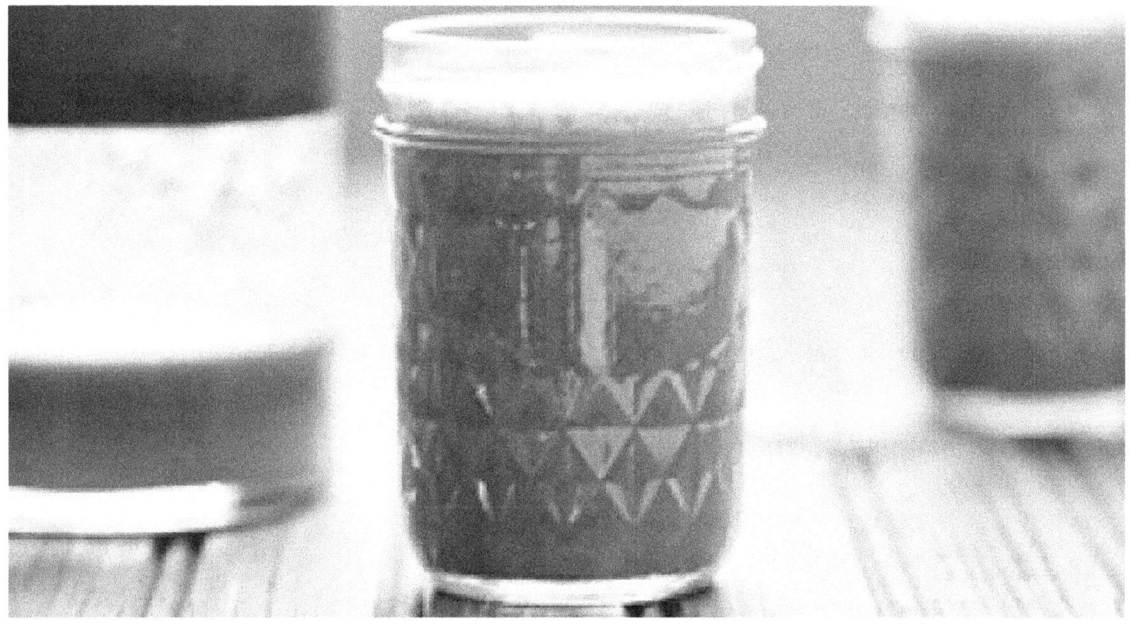

String beans and brussels sprouts are excellent sources of B6, a vitamin that can aid in blood sugar stabilization.

Makes 1 glass (8-ounces)

Serving: 1 glass

Ingredients:

- 10 Organic Brussels sprouts
- 2 Cups organic string beans
- 1 Organic cucumber
- 1 Peeled organic lemon

Directions:

In a juicer, add the Brussels sprouts, string beans, cucumber and the lemon.

Once juiced, pour into a glass lastly and enjoy!

Healthy Heart Juice

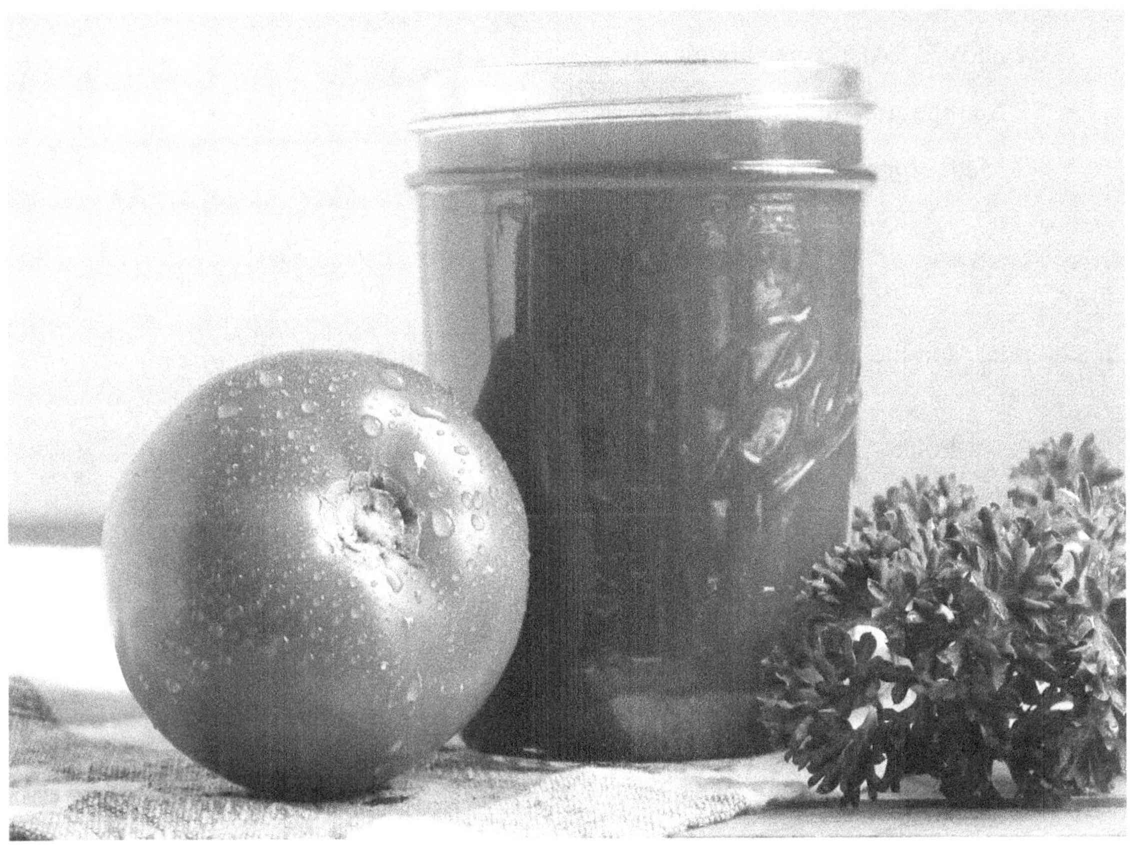

When thinking about how to lower your LDL cholesterol levels, tomatoes, watercress, and apples are the best to pick.

Makes: 1 glass (10-ounces)

Serving: 1 glass

Ingredients:

- 7 Sprigs watercress
- 1 and 1/2 Teaspoons parsley
- 2 Medium tomatoes
- 2 Medium green apples

Directions:

In a blender, add the above ingredients and blend for 1 minute on high.

Pour into a 10-ounce glass and enjoy!

Tropical Mint

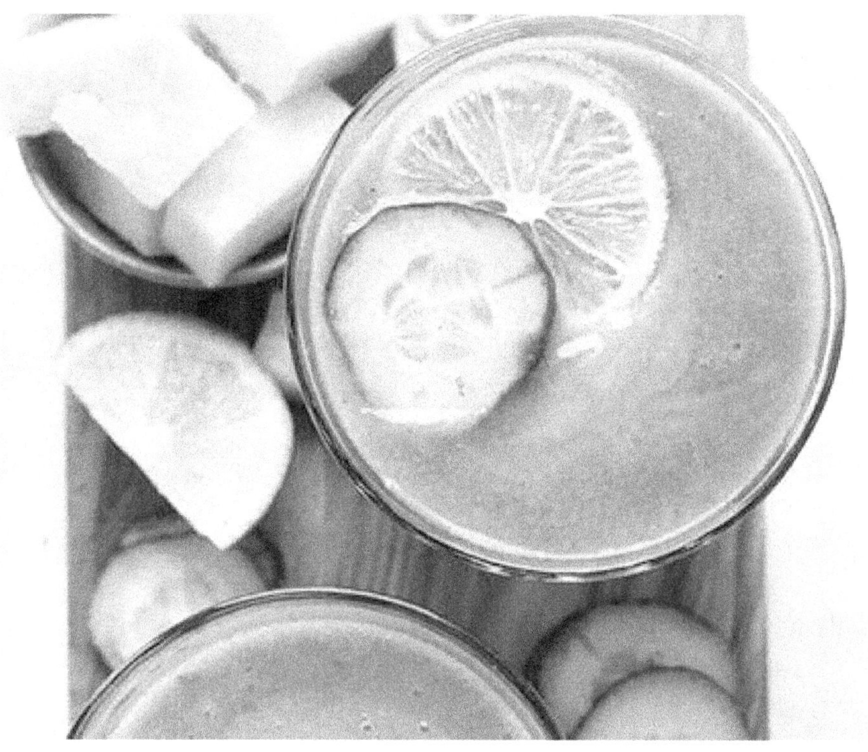

This juice is all most like having a mixed drink. However, this juice will help clean out your whole body.

Makes: 8 cups (8-ounces)

Serving: 1 cup

Ingredients:

- 1 Cup pineapple roughly chopped
- 2 Cups spinach roughly chopped
- 3 Cups whole mint leaves
- 2 Celery stalks
- 1 Small cucumber
- 1 Lemon

Directions:

Place a hard texture first into the juicer, then repeat a soft one until all ingredients have been juiced.

Pour evenly into cups and drink with a loved one.

TIP:

Using fresh cold fruits and vegetables give this juice a nice chill.

Conclusion

I hope this book gives you a new healthier, younger looking body. As you know there are three recipes for the kids. Please use them. And, make sure to check for any food allergies they may have. This goes for the grown-ups all so. Another good point I have to make is there can be side effects to detoxing. Some of them are nausea, headaches, skin rashes, bad breath and chills. This can happen because of your body removing the bad stuff and starting new again.

Best of luck to you own the way to a new you!

About the Author

Ivy's mission is to share her recipes with the world. Even though she is not a professional cook she has always had that flair toward cooking. Her hands create magic. She can make even the simplest recipe tastes superb. Everyone who has tried her food has astounding their compliments was what made her think about writing recipes.

She wanted everyone to have a taste of her creations aside from close family and friends. So, deciding to write recipes was her winning decision. She isn't interested in popularity, but how many people have her recipes reached and touched people. Each recipe in her cookbooks is special and has a special meaning in her life. This means that each recipe is created with attention and love. Every ingredient carefully picked, every combination tried and tested.

Her mission started on her birthday about 9 years ago, when her guests couldn't stop prizing the food on the table. The next thing she did was organizing an event where chefs from restaurants were tasting her recipes. This event gave her the courage to start spreading her recipes.

She has written many cookbooks and she is still working on more. There is no end in the art of cooking; all you need is inspiration, love, and dedication.

Author's Afterthoughts

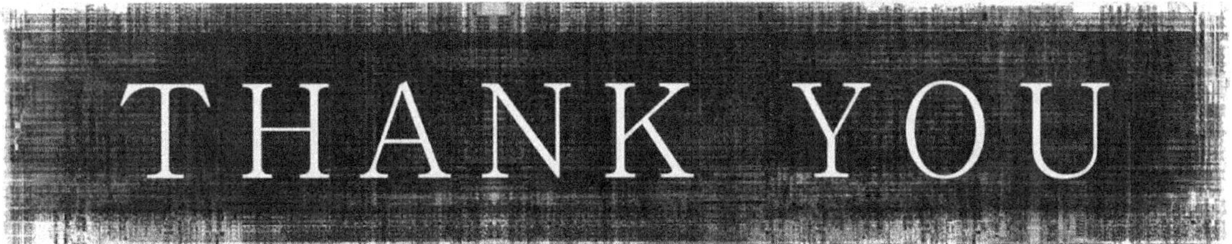

I am thankful for downloading this book and taking the time to read it. I know that you have learned a lot and you had a great time reading it. Writing books is the best way to share the skills I have with your and the best tips too.

I know that there are many books and choosing my book is amazing. I am thankful that you stopped and took time to decide. You made a great decision and I am sure that you enjoyed it.

I will be even happier if you provide honest feedback about my book. Feedbacks helped by growing and they still do. They help me to choose better content and new ideas. So, maybe your feedback can trigger an idea for my next book.

Thank you again

Sincerely

Ivy Hope